MIND
OVER
MENOPAUSE

MIND

OVER
MENOPAUSE

**Lose Weight, Love Your Body,
and Embrace Life After 50 with a
Powerful New Mindset**

PAHLA BOWERS

THE EXPERIMENT

NEW YORK

The Experiment, LLC | 220 East 23rd Street, Suite 600 | New York, NY 10010-4658
theexperimentpublishing.com

The Experiment's books are available at special discounts when purchased in bulk for premiums and sales promotions as well as for fundraising or educational use. For details, contact us at info@theexperimentpublishing.com.

Library of Congress Cataloging-in-Publication Data

Names: Bowers, Pahla, author.
Title: Mind over menopause : lose weight, love your body, and embrace life
   after 50 with a powerful new mindset / Pahla Bowers.
Description: New York : The Experiment, [2023]
Identifiers: LCCN 2023003944 (print) | LCCN 2023003945 (ebook) | ISBN
   9781615199754 (hardcover) | ISBN 9781615199761 (ebook)
Subjects: LCSH: Menopause--Popular works. | Middle aged women--Health and
   hygiene--Popular works. | Older women--Health and hygiene--Popular
   works. | Menopause--Diet therapy--Popular works. | Weight loss--Popular
   works.
Classification: LCC RG186 .B69 2023 (print) | LCC RG186 (ebook) | DDC
   618.1/75--dc23/eng/20230320
LC record available at https://lccn.loc.gov/2023003944
LC ebook record available at https://lccn.loc.gov/2023003945
ISBN 978-1-89101-161-0
Ebook ISBN 978-1-61519-976-1

Cover and text design by Beth Bugler
Cover image (flowers) by happyimages – stock.adobe.com
Author photograph by Tra Huynh (Two Twenty Photos)

Manufactured in the United States of America

First paperback printing May 2024
10 9 8 7 6 5 4 3 2 1

*For Vicki, who never made it to menopause
but would've definitely loved this book*

Contents

INTRODUCTION

~

Well, hello, and welcome to the book. I'm Pahla B, your best middle-aged fitness friend, and I'm here to help you make peace with your menopausal body by using the power of your brain to find a healthy weight, learn to love your body, and embrace the changes of menopause.

No small task, right?

Going through menopause can feel like your whole world is shifting on its axis. Physically, you're suddenly managing somatic symptoms like heart palpitations, sleep disturbances, hot flashes, weight gain, or vaginal dryness. And mentally, you're navigating the grief, anxiety, betrayal, and bewilderment of adapting to your body's changes—all at a time when you might also be experiencing other difficult life transitions like losing your parents, your kids leaving home, a midlife career change, or downsizing your living space.

Menopause isn't *just* about not having your period anymore.

So, What Is Menopause, Anyway?

For many of us, *menopause* is a generic term, covering everything from the moment your periods start getting wonky up until you stop having them. And—like so many female reproductive topics—there's an air of mystery about menopause.

From the time of the ancient Greeks—who thought that a woman's uterus could travel around her body and cause disease—to the near-total medicalization of menopause in the mid-twentieth century to now, it's hard to know what to make of this mid-life change.

In the US, the average age of menopause is fifty-one, and the complete transition from regular cycles to full menopause takes an average of seven years. During the change, over 81 percent of women report one or more somatic symptoms such as hot flashes, night sweats, migraines, or heart palpitations, and 70 percent experience psychological side effects such as anxiety or depression. Medically speaking, there are either two or three distinct phases you go through, and yes, they're defined by your menses (or lack thereof) but include a host of other mental and physical changes, too.

Why two *or* three stages? Because, like many things menopause-related, there's been very little research done, and no medical or scientific community consensus. On the one hand, menopause is significantly more complex and the changes more far-reaching than you might think. And on the other, the disparity in research between men and women, even in modern times, is an area of science that could use improvement.

Here's a timeline of the three-stage model.

- **Perimenopause** starts at the onset of whatever symptoms you may have and lasts up until your final period. Symptoms such as hot flashes, insomnia, and moodiness are happening because your hormones are fluctuating in ways that are different from your usual monthly cycle. Sudden surges, rapid depletion, or lower than usual levels of hormones are presumed to be the cause of most of the symptoms we associate with peri-menopause. While they're troublesome, annoying, inconvenient, and uncomfortable, these symptoms are thankfully not life-threatening, nor are they likely to become chronic.

- **Menopause** is the year after your last period, when you are still quite likely to be experiencing many of the symptoms you had during perimenopause, even though your ovaries have by this point stopped producing estrogen.

- **Postmenopause** is when your menopause has been confirmed, which is twelve months after your last period. Many women experience relief from their physical symptoms at this stage (or soon after), and you might think your physical changes are complete. Unfortunately, this is just the beginning of several serious health risks—specifically heart disease, muscle wasting, cognitive decline, and osteoporosis—that seem to be associated with a lack of estrogen (much more on this in part 3).

The two-stage model makes a slightly different break and avoids using the redundant term *postmenopause* (which, linguistically, is sort of like saying "after-after your last period") while splitting the transition in a way that makes sense with regard to annoying symptoms versus troubling medical risks.

- **Perimenopause** includes everything from the time you begin experiencing any of the symptoms that may be associated with the fluctuation and cessation of your hormones, through the first year (or so—see below) without your period.

- **Menopause** is then the rest of your life, following the confirmation (at twelve months after your last period) of the cessation of your menses.

Of course, this entire "two or three stages" conversation is all assuming that your body got the memo to go through the menopause transition in a linear and orderly fashion. Some of us—I'm raising my hand here—start exhibiting symptoms like anxiety, brain fog, and sleep disturbances in our early forties, while our periods are still pretty regular. And many women will seem to be menopausal and not have a period for several months in a row, then start up again like nothing happened. (Anecdotally, I have a friend who went well over two years without having a period and then had one—hopefully the final one—that was quite a whopper, as though her last egg really wanted to party it up on its way out.)

Thankfully, for our purposes in this book, it's not crucial to be precise about where you are on your personal menopause timeline, though your symptoms aren't irrelevant. There's a good chance those symptoms are affecting you enough that you picked up this book to get some help. More often than not, I'll simply use the word *menopause* to cover the entirety of the menopause transition, while occasionally referring to postmenopause when I want to be clear that it's "after-after" your final period.

No matter what stage of menopause you're currently experiencing, your body has already changed, it is currently changing, and—due to the aging process as much as menopause—it will continue to change for the rest of your life. For many of us, accepting these changes feels *hard*, so I've written this book to help you change your mind about that.

A Quick Word about Hormone Replacement Therapy

Since it might be on your mind right about now, I want to clarify that I'm not a doctor, and any conversation about hormone replacement therapy is above my pay grade. There are definitely pros and cons to taking hormones to relieve your menopausal symptoms, but helping you make that decision is well beyond the scope of this book.

In full transparency, I am not currently taking any estrogen therapy, but I do have a progestin-releasing IUD to help curtail heavy menstrual bleeding (nothing like a little TMI right here in the introduction to the book, right?). While I have plenty of personal opinions about hormones and doctors and pharmaceutical companies, they're not relevant for this book. I truly believe that the best decision about hormone treatment for you is the one you arrive at, armed with information from your own body and discussed with your health care provider.

Some Clarification about the Words *Estrogen* and *Hormones*

Throughout this book, I'll be using the word *hormones* in a very general way to refer to the chemicals your body produces in order to regulate thousands of different bodily processes. The intricacies of how hormones work together is well beyond the scope of this book, and the information is only offered to give you a broad idea of how your body works. I'll also be using the word *estrogen* as though it's one thing, but it's actually at least three separate-but-related hormones. This book is not intended as medical advice, nor is it meant to be a science textbook with a thorough explanation of the complexities of the hormonal changes of menopause. Rather, I'm offering you a big-picture view of what's going on in your body, with reassurance that you feel different now because you *are* different. When your body stops producing estrogen(s), it fundamentally affects all of your systems, your bodily processes, and your mind.

Further, you'll notice that I don't mention progesterone—which is also a singular form used generically to describe a group of related hormones and their synthetic counterparts—as significantly impacting menopause, even though your body will also stop production of progesterone as it stops making estrogen. The current medical knowledge suggests that progesterone is a "pro-gestation" hormone, meaning that its major function is related to the temporary conditions of pregnancy and childbirth. Therefore, the cessation of production isn't likely to be problematic or cause noticeable changes for menopausal women. In fact, many of symptoms of premenstrual syndrome (PMS) are attributed to progesterone, so you might even feel less moody, bloated, or tender after menopause when you're not producing it anymore.

Who Am I to Be Telling You What to Think about Menopause?

Well, truthfully, I'm *not* going to tell you what to think, though I will make a few friendly suggestions throughout this book. Far more effective than simply handing you some happy thoughts that may or may not work for you and sending you on your way to muddle through on your own, I'm going to show you exactly how to find your best (and worst) thoughts for yourself. And my expertise on this comes first and foremost from my own experience.

I'm a certified life coach, an ultramarathoner, an entrepreneur, a YouTube fitness instructor, the mother of two grown men that I still refer to as "my boys," and a woman in the middle of the glorious menopause transition myself. I've had an up-close-and-personal view of what changing hormones have done to my athletic body, my mental clarity, my stamina, my self-esteem, and my waistline. I have felt the despair of hormonal changes I didn't understand, and I have pulled myself out of it by doing the exact work I am describing for you in this book.

Oh, and I also hold several physical and mental health certifications (Personal Trainer, Functional Fitness Specialist, Health Coach, and Life and Weight Coach) and have a decade and a half of experience working with women who want to lose weight and/or create positive change in their lives.

Very early in my fitness career—when I was still a mere forty years old and didn't have a clue what menopause held in store for me—I worked for a popular chain of group fitness centers that were known for their clientele of a "certain age." I didn't love the job because I'm better suited to being my own boss, but I sure loved the women who came in to exercise every day. A few years later, when I was out on my own as an in-home personal trainer, I had the great privilege of being invited into the living rooms of dozens of menopausal women (my first client was my then seventy-year-old mom). The stories I heard and the insights I gained about their unique menopause-related weight loss and fitness struggles deeply informed the kind of coach I am today.

Making the leap from in-home personal training to creating online workout videos on YouTube and coaching inside my Get Your Goal group membership has earned me the amazing pleasure of helping thousands of women lose many thousands of pounds and learn to love exercising while making peace with their menopausal bodies. Even though I don't exercise with any of my clients personally anymore, I'm still grateful to be considered part of their daily routines. Through the magic of the internet, I can and share your trials and your successes.

In the course of my life and my fitness career, I've seen a lot of bodies of all ages, shapes, and sizes. I've recorded a lot of weights, body fat percentages, and waist measurements. As both a fitness professional and professional life coach, I've been gifted with deeply personal stories that will never see the light of day, and I have witnessed some fantastic success stories that I will share here in this book (with names and identifying details changed).

The most profound lesson I've learned through my own experience, and in working with other women is this: **Your body responds to what your brain believes.** There is no way to escape this fundamental truth—and that's great news! Because it means that if you want to change your body, you need to start with changing your mindset. And not only do I know exactly how to do that, but I can teach you to do it, too.

Understanding Your Mindset

One of the ways I like to think about mindset is to picture an overnight bag full of your chosen outfits and shoes, toiletry essentials, nightwear, assorted electronics chargers, medicines, a change (or three) of underclothes, and a "just in case we go somewhere fancy" outfit. When you take that bag with you on a quick weekend getaway, it has everything you need to enjoy yourself.

But what if your flight lands you at a completely unexpected destination? And instead of putting on your walking shoes and extra sunscreen for a day at Disneyland, you're randomly required to attend a gala fundraiser with celebrities and politicians? Now, all of a sudden, the items you've packed are completely inappropriate (except for that "just in case" outfit—thank goodness you grabbed that at the last minute).

The individual shirts and jeans and hats you packed lovingly into your luggage are your *beliefs*—thoughts you have about yourself, your body, and your ability to lose weight or navigate changes. Together, zipped into your cute traveling bag, this collection of thoughts is your *mindset*.

Your mindset is neither good nor bad, and it doesn't mean anything about you that your luggage doesn't meet the needs of your vacation. When you packed that bag, you had the full expectation of using each item and having a good time at your planned destination. But when you wound up somewhere else, it turned out that the clothing and supplies you brought weren't useful to you. That's not the problem of your overnight bag, nor was it intentionally bad planning on your part. It just . . . *is*.

Now, hopefully you've never experienced a vacation quite as unexpected as this, but as an analogy, this one's spot on. You have arrived here at menopause, which can sure feel like a tropical island sometimes, with luggage that was packed for an Alaskan cruise.

But here's the best news of all: It turns out that your overnight bag has a magical false bottom with an *unending supply* of useful garments, and even the clothes and shoes you did bring might not be as inappropriate for this location as you feared. Together throughout this book, we're going to take a look at your shirts, your shorts, and your shoes and decide which ones to keep in the bag, so you can still enjoy a dream vacation.

How to Change Your Mind
(about Menopause or Anything Else)

We're going to spend a fair bit of time in this book exploring how your thoughts and feelings work, so let me take a quick moment here to be clear that I am not a psychiatrist, doctor, or scientist, nor is this book trying to explain brain science, metabolism, exercise science, or your hormones in anything other than layperson's terms.

The foundation of my mindset assertions in this book lie in cognitive behavioral therapy (CBT)—a well-studied and widely used psychotherapy protocol, which, at its heart, helps people change their behaviors by challenging the veracity of their thoughts. The roots of CBT go all the way back to ancient Stoic philosophers but have been honed in the last fifty years or so as psychologists merged two differing schools of thought about how the mind works—behaviorism and cognition—into one, with documented success in treating depression and anxiety. Now, the tools used for CBT are making their way into the mainstream through life coaching. Here are the basic tenets of CBT, how they work, and how we'll apply them in this book.

- **Your thoughts create your feelings and your feelings drive your actions.** This is a big one, and both parts are counterintuitive to what we're taught socially. The way we typically speak about our thoughts and feelings reflects a belief that other people, outside forces, and things that happen in the world make us feel things ("Traffic was so frustrating on my commute this morning!"), but this is not true. Our thoughts quite literally—through the magic of biology that is your personal hormonal and chemical makeup—*create* our feelings. We also tend to believe that we have the ability to do things solely because we want or decide to do them. This is only partially true—we can definitely make ourselves do things in the short term through willpower, but over any length of time, our feelings-driven brain will revert to its natural way of dictating our behaviors. Which is to say, your feelings drive your actions.

- **When you question the truth of your thoughts, you open the door to other outcomes.** This is the seed of every change you might want to make in your life: Simply recognize that what you think right now might not be the truth, and it is not the only possibility of what you could think. This is one of the most powerful principles you will ever realize, and it's *the* idea that leads to every personal transformation—because if you think something different, you'll feel different, which will lead to different actions, and therefore different outcomes.

- **Your thoughts (and therefore, your feelings and actions) are either moving you toward your goal or away from it.** This is the crux of what I'll be teaching you in this book, and I've created an incredibly useful tool that will help you understand which of your thoughts are leading you in which direction.

How to Use this Book

First, I encourage you to have an open mind about the concepts I'll be teaching you, because so many of them are going to sound counterintuitive if this is your first exposure to them. I'm literally going to tell you that "eating less and moving more" is *causing* your menopausal weight gain, for example. What this might mean for you is that you'll want to read it in small doses rather than plowing through the whole book at once. But on the other hand, maybe you learn best by getting the "big picture" first and then coming back for the details.

Truly, both ways will get you where you want to go, and taking a quick second right now to decide for yourself and then trust your decision illustrates one of the main concepts I want to offer you: You have the power (and the permission) to do this work *your* way, which will therefore become the *best* way (and the *right* way) to reach your goals.

This concept of doing things your own way can be one of the biggest stumbling blocks for women on a quest to lose weight. You're told constantly by the fitness and diet industry that if you're not doing things their way or getting the results you've been promised, it must be because *you're* doing something wrong. Rather than viewing your progress through the lens of "right" or "wrong," I encourage you to see all your experiences—no matter the results they created—as opportunities to learn the next thing that will propel you forward to success.

And then, finally, you'll be most successful with this book if you come at the work as though it's a skill you're learning, because it is. Make no mistake, there's *work* to be done here; changing your mind about menopause isn't going to just happen by itself. It's not just reading and passively intellectualizing the material that will create change in your life. You will need to physically practice the skill to get any traction with it, and you're liable to be sort of bad—or at least awkward—at it when you get started. That is not only okay but expected, and it does not in any way indicate that you aren't going to be great at it in the future. You are.

If you were already good at any of this, you wouldn't need this book. And that's why I wrote it: So you're not alone and struggling to figure this out for yourself. I've got you.

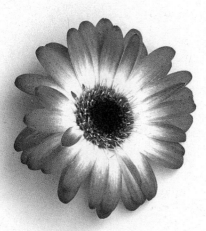

PART ONE

The Power of Your Brain

CHAPTER 1

The Key That Unlocks Every Door

Menopause Has Changed Your Body, So It's Time for You to Change Your Mind

Welcome to menopause, where everything you thought you knew about your body changed overnight. You're always hot (unless of course you're freezing cold), you're moodier than ever, sleep seems like a distant memory, and all that sunbathing you did in your teens and twenties is showing up in the form of "age spots" and skin like crepe paper. It's as though you turned fifty and the world you lived in during your thirties and forties is just *gone*—your kids grew up, your parents became elderly, your friends started retiring, and suddenly your body feels like a complete mystery to you.

You've been slashing your calories and cranking up the cardio, but somehow your pants are still getting tighter. Your muscles have gone from taut and toned to soft and saggy, and no matter how many sit-ups you do, that *meno-pot* is mocking you in the full-length mirror. Your friends agree that menopause is the worst, and your doctor's best advice is to just accept that weight gain is inevitable at your age. You can't help but wonder, is this it? Is this midlife—full of misery, frustration, and belly fat?

Thankfully, no.

This is only a pit stop on your way to a brilliant second half, where you find your way to a healthy weight, break free from years of diet restriction, and finally make peace with your beautifully changing menopausal body. Right now, you're about to figure it out and live happily ever after. And that's why I'm here, playing the role of the savvy friend who's already worked through these feeling and changes—plus done enough scientific reading to understand some of the biology of what's going on—to help you make peace with menopause.

The road ahead of you might seem frightening right now, but it's actually an exciting one, where you get to challenge all the paradigms that shaped your premenopausal life, decide where you want to go next, and intentionally create what your life will look like when you get there. Because not only are you not a victim of biology, it is the source of your greatest power.

How I Got Here: My Menopause and Mindset Story

A few years ago, when I was in my late forties, I was enjoying what I now recognize as the peak of my middle-aged fitness—running long distances with ease and maintaining a thin, strong body without thinking too hard about it. Right about that same time, as my kids were graduating from high school and my periods were becoming wildly unpredictable, my older sister Vicki (who was my best friend) was diagnosed with cancer and died just six and a half months later.

Being a fitness trainer and an avid runner, I reacted to my grief, my change of status as a working stay-at-home mom, and my fear of impending menopausal changes by doing something that sounded completely rational at the time: I signed up to run a 110K ultramarathon (that's 68 miles of running for my nonmetric friends). I was attempting to run away from my sadness, my worries, and a lot of confusion about my life, and I truly believed that throwing myself into the sport I'd loved for years would help me to "feel like myself again."

Instead, it was just the opposite—I found myself getting tired and easily overwhelmed, I battled constant minor aches and injuries, and I started gaining weight.

Don't get me wrong, I didn't pack on fifty pounds overnight. It was more like ten pounds over the course of six months. Honestly, many women might not have even noticed a small gain like this, but it was concerning for me as a fitness professional and as a woman who had spent more than a dozen years feeling impervious to weight struggles.

For a while, I tried to convince myself that the weight gain was temporary and told myself that of course I could just take it off easily when I wanted to. But then, when I was ready to lose those pesky pounds, they didn't come off the way I'd expected. I tried eating less, even though I wasn't eating very much. I tried exercising even more, in spite of already exercising quite a bit. And rather than seeing the scale trend downward, it kept climbing.

So, I did what lots of us do in situations like these: I completely ignored how lousy I felt and doubled down on all the things I was doing that weren't working.

After that 110K run, I signed up for five more ultramarathons over the next eleven months, and that did not work out well for me. I was definitely moving more and eating less, but I not only didn't lose any weight, I had frequent headaches, I was often crabby or out of sorts, my sleep was disrupted, and my appetite was nonexistent. I was verging on both emotional and physical exhaustion and had no idea what to do about it, because I hadn't faced hormonal changes like these since I was a teenager (and I didn't handle it well then, either).

So many women chalk these symptoms up to menopause and feel like we just have to grit our teeth and get through it. The prevailing wisdom from my friends and family was that getting older means gaining weight, losing fitness, and feeling lousy most of the time, so why should I be any different?

Because I *wanted* to be different. I wanted to keep loving my body the way I had for years, and to feel good about myself—even during menopause.

As an exercise coach, I am passionate about understanding how the human body moves and—even beyond my professional experience—I'm also very curious about *why* it does the things it does. So, in pursuit of losing a few pounds (while training for an ultramarathon, of course), off I went to the internet, to gain some insight into why my menopausal body seemed unable to lose weight in ways that had worked for me in my twenties, thirties, and most of my forties.

What I found was a lot of people trying to convince me that intermittent fasting or a keto diet were the only ways to lose weight in my fifties.

As an athlete, fitness trainer, and endurance runner, I've spent the better part of two decades ignoring the low-carb craze, because—to put it bluntly—it simply doesn't apply to me. Athletic performance requires frequent, nearly constant replenishment of fuel, and the fuel most readily available to the human body for energetic movement comes from carbohydrates. Neither keto nor intermittent fasting would meet my needs. So, I continued my search.

Again and again, the only information I could find about weight loss for women over fifty seemed to focus solely on eating in specific (not ultramarathon- or even exercise-friendly) ways. I realized then that maybe I was asking Google the wrong question. Yes, I wanted to lose weight, but I also wanted to keep running and working out at the level I'd been accustomed to. Why couldn't my menopausal body hold a steady weight and handle exercise the way it used to?

By positioning my question as a problem with athletic training, I hit the information jackpot and found a handful of studies linking the lower estrogen levels of menopausal women with prolonged exercise recovery times (which, by proxy, spurs weight gain). I was simultaneously thrilled to find this information—it explained everything I'd been feeling and noticing in my own body—and absolutely devastated by what it meant for me as a woman who loves to run long distances for fun.

The information was clear, and I understood intellectually that I needed to rein in my running in order to achieve my weight loss goal. But emotionally I was crushed while trying to come to terms with what felt like another huge loss in my life.

In February 2020, I ran what was likely my final ultramarathon and committed myself fully to the daily tasks of weigh-loss: eating properly, hydrating, sleeping, and exercising moderately. I physically curtailed my workouts and started to see results on the scale, but the daily battle inside my head about wanting to exercise as much as I was used to was exhausting. After months of gritting my teeth and trying to "get through this," I finally realized that what I wanted— much more than weight loss—was to feel good; not just to weigh a certain number, but to really feel happy and loving toward my life and my body. This new, "whole body and mind" goal meant that it was time to step out of my *dieting* mentality, start paying attention to the way I was speaking to myself, get curious about why I wanted to exercise so much, figure out how to listen to the signals my body was sending me, and finally explore my grief.

It was time to look inside my brain and see what was going on in there that was keeping me stuck and miserable in a body and a life I didn't recognize. This is a book about your body, for sure— as a weight loss and exercise expert, I have lots of practical, scientific information to share that will help you make sense of your miraculously changing biology—but even more important, it's a book about changing your mindset to make the most of your menopause.

How understanding my brain changed everything

I started my mindset journey many years ago not by working on weight-loss but rather on my thoughts about money. At the time, I was what I would refer to as a "chronic underearner," with dozens of unhelpful beliefs about my ability to make money, save money, keep money, and spend money. I had already been sorting through those money mindset blocks for a few years, with only limited success.

I had started my own in-home personal training business in 2012 and then added making online fitness videos and posting them to YouTube in 2013. Between the constant driving to client's houses, creation of workouts, filming, editing, social media posting, advertising, and bookkeeping, I was working more than full-time hours. And yet, even after five years of steadily increasing my clients and my viewership, my annual gross income in 2017 hovered at just over $5,000. After expenses, I was actually losing money at my job!

But in the weird way that things sometimes work themselves out, in 2019, when I went looking for resources to help me with my grief after my sister died, I ended up finding a podcast called *The Life Coach School* (by Brooke Castillo) that would change my entire life. In just a few months of binge-listening to nearly every episode, I started to ease my sadness, dramatically increase my income, improve my relationships, and change my body. And just two years later, after certifying as a Life and Weight Coach (through the Life Coach School), the happy accident of finding that podcast set me on the course to an even more satisfying career than I had ever imagined for myself.

By way of *The Life Coach School* podcast, I was introduced to the principles of cognitive behavioral therapy that I'll be sharing with you in this book. Hearing the principles of growth mindset, positive psychology, and the Law of Attraction explained through the lens of biology, evolution, and brain science was what finally clicked things into place for me in a way that nothing else could. After years of "trying to work on my mindset," I was amazed to discover that once I understood and accepted how and why my brain behaved the way it did, I wasn't "trying" to create positive changes in my life anymore. I was actually *doing* it.

Where I've used CBT in my life, and how it can help you, too

I started listening to *The Life Coach School* podcast in January 2019 for the express purpose of managing and alleviating my grief. But not long into listening, I discovered a treasure trove of helpful information about uncovering my money blocks and creating a more lucrative and satisfying business. As I mentioned, my gross income in 2017 was around $5,000, but the next year was significantly better at just over $16,000. By the end of 2019, I had generated a gross income of over $40,000—the most money I'd ever made in one year in my entire life. I vividly remember doing the math and crying tears of disbelief and joy when I saw that number. It was the first tangible evidence I had that I could *actually* create anything I wanted in my life. Yes, I had been listening to podcasts and reading books and watching YouTube videos from people who all said it would work this way—that your thoughts create your reality—but here were *my* thoughts creating *my* reality and proving it true! It felt mind-blowing.

So, of course I had to test it in other areas, because it couldn't be that simple, right? But it was.

At first, I didn't even realize how much I was internalizing the ideas and concepts of CBT. But after my success with money, I turned my intention to improving my relationships with family members, and quickly recognized that I had unrealistic and unhelpful expectations of other people that were creating constant low-grade feelings of stress and resentment for me. Once I started focusing my attention on creating feelings of love and compassion—for myself and my family members—so many of my negative emotions began to melt away. With my *thoughts*, I created the *reality* of loving relationships.

Coming to terms with the grief of losing my sister has been the most challenging and worthwhile work I've ever done, and I would consider it an ongoing process. It's a very different goal than wanting to make a certain amount of money in a year. But when I got started, I felt passionately that I didn't want to remain stuck in my grief, and I knew that was going to take effort on my part. The fact of my sister's passing coinciding with my menopause transition might seem unfortunate, but for me, it was truly the best timing I could have asked for. Processing the grief I felt over my changing body melded into the grief I felt about losing my best friend and made clear where I was thinking and feeling in unhelpful ways. And the end result for both relationships is the same—I love my sister, even though she's gone, and I love my body, even though it's different now, too. With my *thoughts*, I created the *reality* of acceptance and peace.

Let me be really clear that, first, listening to a podcast and using cognitive behavioral therapy tools didn't magically "fix" things in my life, and second, creating success is not just a matter of thinking good thoughts to bring good things into my life. In fact, it's nearly the opposite on both of those points! Yes, I make more money, have satisfying relationships, and feel at peace with my sister's death as well as with my changing menopausal body—and, simultaneously, I still struggle with all these things. Old thoughts will surface, my husband will say or do something that I think is annoying, or I'll get hit with a grief bomb when a song I haven't heard in a long time comes on the radio.

There's not going to be a time in my life when I never think about money again, or don't have knee-jerk reactions to situations, or stop mourning my losses. The difference—and the difference you can create, too—is that rather than being flummoxed by the bad feelings, I welcome them. This is what I mean when I say that you don't create good results in your life just by thinking good thoughts. You're far better served by accepting, allowing, and being unafraid of the bad thoughts, too.

If I had to pick the thing that's missing from many of the self-help books I've read, it's this: On your way to feeling better and thinking positive thoughts, you're also going to feel lousy and need to acknowledge and work with your negative thoughts. That might sound like a tough pill to swallow right now, but I promise you, it's a very low price to pay for what you'll get in return. With practice, a bit of bravery to look at your thoughts and feelings head-on, and the simple formula I'm about to share with you (the key to making the magic happen), you will be able to create the reality *you* want in *your* life.

The Two-Step Tool

Let's get started on creating the reality you want to see in your life with step-by-step instructions that are easy to follow and work every time. In order to improve your relationship with your weight, your body, and your journey through menopause, you're going to use an incredibly simple formula that I call the Two-Step Tool. Here's what it looks like.

- Step One is to **find your thoughts.**
- Step Two is to **decide if they're helpful.**

If this sounds easy, that's because it is! But don't let the simplicity fool you. When I initially created this tool, I didn't entirely understand how powerful it was, so first, let me show you what the Two-Step Tool does and how it works, and then I'll explain exactly how to use it.

What the Two-Step Tool does

Every single thought you have is creating a result in your life. We all have lots and lots of thoughts—about sixty thousand a day—and we don't hear most of them. According to cognitive neuroscientists, we are only aware of about 5 percent of our thoughts. But all day long, your unheard and unnoticed thoughts are in the background, ruling your life and shaping your reality through a chain of events that, in all likelihood, you rarely take the time to pay attention to. It goes like this.

You have a thought and it creates a feeling. A thought is an electric impulse in your brain that sets off a chemical reaction of hormones that results in physiological responses in your body—things like an elevated heart rate, a sweat response, and shallow breathing, to name a few. Through years of social conditioning and vocabulary building, you've learned to identify those sensations with labels like fear, happiness, stress, or excitement—emotion words. Even the thoughts that you don't hear consciously are creating these subtle and sometimes not-so-subtle vibrations in your body. This is why you'll sometimes find yourself in a bad mood and not know why. Your brain is doing exactly what brains do—thinking thoughts and creating feelings!

That feeling drives actions (and inactions). When you have that physical vibration in your body (even if you don't notice it consciously), you respond by behaving in certain ways. Good feelings like happiness, excitement, or motivation will cause you to act with energy—speaking confidently, being productive, imagining a rosy future, and reliving past successes, for example—and not acting in ways that would hamper your success. Bad feelings such as anger, sadness, fear, or boredom will drive actions that are not likely in your best interests. When you've had the physical vibrations associated with a bad feeling, you've probably noticed yourself snapping at others, avoiding important tasks, eating to comfort yourself, or mindlessly shopping online from your work desk.

Those actions (and inactions) create results in your life. And finally, this (sometimes incredibly quick, blink-and-you-missed-it) chain of events culminates in creating results in your life that are a direct reflection of your original thought. Therefore, if there is a result you want for yourself that you don't already have—such as weighing an amount you don't already weigh—that simply means you are having thoughts right now that are creating your current weight rather than your desired weight.

For example, let's imagine a situation where you're reading a weight-loss book like this one, and you had the fleeting thought "I'm never going to lose weight," which created a sinking feeling in your stomach and a heavy heart that—if you noticed it at all—you would call dread. When you felt that dread—even if you didn't consciously recognize feeling it—about your inability to lose weight successfully, you probably started to ruminate over past failures, or imagined a worst-case scenario outcome of gaining even more weight. You might also have tried to escape the feeling of dread—which you still might not have recognized or named!—by getting something to eat or checking social media on your phone. Thinking, worrying, and distracting yourself are all *actions* that were directly driven from the feeling of dread—even if you never recognized yourself feeling it.

Additionally, because the feeling of dread is uncomfortable for most of us, you might also have attempted to ignore or avoid it by putting the book down or not familiarizing yourself with the skills you need to develop for success—these are *inactions*. And when you see it all laid out like this, it's clear that the thought "I'm never going to lose weight" directly *created* the result of "never" losing weight.

Conversely, a thought like "I'm terrific at losing weight" would create weight-loss success because that thought would spark a feeling of excitement, which would drive actions like finishing this book, imagining future success, being thoroughly prepared, and not wasting time on your phone. In other words, your *thought* about being terrific at weight loss would create terrific weight-loss *results*.

The Two-Step Tool will help you sort through what you're thinking and find the unhelpful thoughts that are producing the results you don't want (such as your current weight) as well as the helpful thoughts that will produce the result you do want (your goal weight). It helps you see your thoughts clearly and categorize them in a way that's incredibly powerful to your brain and moves you forward toward your goal.

I like to think of it as a crime scene investigation, and now feels like a good time to mention that I have a bachelor of science degree in criminology, earned at a time in my life (the mid-1990s) when I really thought I was going to be a detective for the FBI like Dana Scully from *The X-Files*. I have a deep fascination with knowing how and why things have happened, which I've never used in a law enforcement setting but which serves me better than you might think as a life coach.

If you've ever watched a show like *Forensic Files* (which is very different from *The X-Files*), you've seen how sometimes the place where a crime has been committed has been cleaned up by the perpetrator, right? And then, like magic, the crime scene technicians come in with a black light and find all the hidden traces of blood? This is exactly what the Two-Step Tool does! It takes a situation where you can't necessarily see your thoughts and it illuminates the areas where there's evidence of an unhelpful thought and where there's not.

So, when you're using the Two-Step Tool and you find an unhelpful thought, you can simply imagine it glowing in the dark like traces of dried blood, spelling out the words "This thought won't get you where you want to go!"

Just Thinking Good Thoughts Isn't the Answer

When I first heard that your thoughts create your reality, it seemed that the answer to getting everything I wanted in life was pretty simple: Just think good thoughts.

Unfortunately, not quite. Sitting around thinking good thoughts doesn't get any work done toward your goals. Aha! So, the answer is still pretty simple: Just think good thoughts and do the right things.

Nope, we're still not there. The reason your *thoughts* create your reality is because of the middle link in the chain—your *feelings*. All three components—thought, feeling, and action—have to be present, and this is why neither affirmations (thoughts) nor willpower (actions) alone can get you all the way to your goals. You can force yourself to think good thoughts, and you can force yourself to do things, but you can't force your feelings.

What the Two-Step Tool *doesn't* do

Many of us come to mindset work thinking that we need to solve a problem, such as how to lose weight—something that's on our minds and bothering us today. We believe that coming to conclusions and resolving that particular issue will make us feel better right now. And then, because we feel better, *everything* in our lives will magically be better.

The truth is that, yes, over time and with consistent use of the Two-Step Tool, you will be able to solve problems and you will feel better, but these are gradual processes rather than the product of any single instance of thinking about your thoughts and deciding if they're helpful.

Instead, each time you do this work, what you'll come away with is *self-awareness*.

Right now that might sound like receiving socks for your birthday when you were a kid, but self-awareness is better than the newest, coolest toy. It's the greatest gift you can give yourself because self-awareness is the unskippable foundation—like learning the alphabet before you can read—of creating intentional change in your life.

When you become aware of the thoughts you're thinking and can see clearly that they're not helpful in reaching your goals, you will hold the key that unlocks the door to your success.

How to use the Two-Step Tool in real life

Step One of the Two-Step Tool is to find your thoughts, which is to say, "write stuff down in your journal."

Ugh, Pahla, there's absolutely no way that journaling is going to help me lose weight!

I completely get it—Oprah told you that journaling was helpful, so you tried writing down your thoughts, but it either felt like you were just writing a list of what you did today, or else it seemed like you were doing a lot of complaining on paper. Or maybe you've never tried journaling before because it sounded too intimidating, or painfully boring, or something in between, and frankly, you just don't see what the fuss is about.

Well, the reason journaling never felt useful before—that is, if you journaled at all—is because it *wasn't*. Simply writing things down is *nice*, and sometimes it helps you get things off your chest. In fact, sometimes you might even feel like you've solved a problem or made yourself feel better. But without the second step of the Two-Step Tool—which, combined with Step One, is how you get *self-awareness*—you're not propelling yourself toward your goals.

Step Two of the Two-Step Tool is to decide if each of those thoughts you've found is helpful, and here's how: Ask yourself how you *feel* when you think them.

Seriously, Pahla? What do my feelings have to do with it?

In a word: EVERYTHING.

You are a feelings-driven creature, simply by virtue of being a mammal with an instinctive drive to seek pleasure and avoid pain.

Want to see this in action? Here's a question for you: *Why do you want to lose weight?*

So you can be healthy. Awesome. *Why do you want to be healthy?*

So you can live a long life. Excellent. *Why do you want to live a long life?*

So you can enjoy time with your family and friends and not die young. Ah, yes, also known as "seeking pleasure and avoiding pain."

Everything you want in life, from large-scale dreams like building a million-dollar business or losing a hundred pounds to "small stuff" like putting on fuzzy socks when it's cold in your house, is some version of pleasure—and this is good news! When it comes to deciding if your thoughts are helpful in reaching your goal, it means that you have an incredible, foolproof compass built directly into your body that can point you exactly where you want to go.

When you find a thought about your goal and that thought feels GOOD—such as happy, excited, motivated, energized, creative, inspired, thrilled, loving, calm, powerful, self-assured, eager, playful, secure, focused, healthy, trusting, ambitious, brave, capable, satisfied, relaxed, proud, free, or courageous—then that thought is HELPFUL, because good feelings drive "good"* actions. And good actions—such as eating properly, drinking your water, sleeping well, and exercising appropriately—will get you the good results (in this example, weight loss) that you're aiming for.

If you have a thought about your goal and it feels BAD—such as angry, sad, reluctant, trapped, lost, disgusted, irritated, stressed, depleted, helpless, resentful, dejected, unworthy, jealous, lonely, ashamed, unhappy, defeated, embarrassed, miserable, resigned, hesitant, furious, anxious, or overwhelmed—then that thought is UNHELPFUL, because bad feelings drive "bad" actions. Bad actions, inactions, and avoidance behaviors—such as emotional eating, skipping your water, staying up too late, or over-exercising—will stall or even stop your progress toward your goal.

How to Use the Two-Step Tool in Seven Very Detailed Steps

While the Two-Step Tool is, at its heart, an incredibly simple journaling technique that yields a bounty of self-awareness, there are also some nuances to each step that will help you use it successfully that I'm going to outline for you here before you put it to use in the next chapter. Don't get lost in the weeds, though—when you're struggling to find self-awareness, remember that it always comes down to the basics of finding your thoughts and deciding if they're helpful.

---

* A note about the quotation marks around *good* and *bad* in the above discussion: Truly, there's no such thing as good or bad thoughts, or feelings, or actions. All thoughts, all feelings, and all actions are part of our gloriously messy and amazingly weird human experience. However, for the specific purpose of getting to your desired goal, some thoughts, feelings, and actions will help you get there and others won't. Hence my use of the words *helpful* and *unhelpful* throughout this book.

Here's exactly how to journal with the Two-Step Tool.

1. Ask yourself a direct and specific question.

2. Write down everything that pops into your head.

3. Put the phrase "I think" in front of each sentence.

4. Listen to each sentence and notice what feeling the thought creates for you.

5. Decide if the feeling for that thought is good or bad.

6. Write "Unhelpful" next to each thought that feels bad and "Helpful" next to the ones that feel good.

7. Let your brain do the rest of the work.

Ask yourself a direct and specific question

Your brain always wants to answer a question, and you can use this to your advantage with the Two-Step Tool. This quirk of your brain is evidence of evolution at work: Our ancestors who could solve problems—that is, answer a question—were the ones who survived, and this trait is so strong in the modern human brain that it feels instinctive. Fun fact: Advertisers take advantage of this compulsion all the time to attract your attention by asking a question at the beginning of an ad. Have you noticed this before? (See how you wanted to answer me? It works!) Asking yourself a question will catch your brain's attention and get your thoughts flowing. Here's a pro tip: Start your question with "What do I think about . . . ?" and strive to ask yourself something direct, specific, and as nonjudgmental as possible. For example, a question like "What do I think about the number of calories I ate today?" will yield self-awareness better than "What's wrong with me?" Throughout this book, I offer you ideas for journal prompts that you can use exactly as they are, or with your own personal spin. Even the act of choosing a question can be an opportunity for self-awareness.

Write down everything that pops into your head

Writing down everything you think, exactly the way you think it, is tougher than it sounds. This is partially because your thoughts are fast-moving (sixty thousand thoughts a day means you're thinking nearly a thought every second), but also because you're likely to want to censor yourself in some manner. Wanting to write down a sanitized version of your thoughts is super common and can be overcome once you're aware of it. Many of us—at least unconsciously—don't want to be thinking negative thoughts, or worry that somebody else might read our words, or believe that writing them down makes our thoughts more "real" in some way. But in fact, getting your thoughts down on paper will have the opposite effect and will help you gain agency over them and develop trust in yourself. Creating a nonjudgmental journaling space is the foundation for self-awareness, and—not coincidentally—will be the thing that helps you change your thoughts in the long run. If this step proves to be difficult for any reason—some of us immediately freeze up in the face of a blank piece of paper—offer yourself an actionable standard to meet, such as finding just one or two thoughts. And, of course, if you have concerns about privacy, feel free to shred your journal pages when you're done with them or lock them inside a password-protected document on your computer.

Put the phrase "I think" in front of each sentence

The simple act of writing "I think" at the beginning of each of your thoughts is a step in the direction of changing them, because it will help your brain recognize that they are thoughts instead of facts. From a practical journaling standpoint, this might mean rewriting your thoughts on another piece of paper, or simply leaving yourself the space for this addendum when you get started. Personally, I like to write each thought on a separate line in my journal as it's coming out of my head, then go back and write "I think" in front of each one after I've finished. Alternatively, you can also just say to yourself "I think . . ." when you're completing the next step. As long as you've taken the time and space to recognize that every sentence is a *thought*—rather than a fact or a truth—you're doing this step correctly.

Listen to each sentence and notice what feeling the thought creates for you

Your thought is a tiny spark of electricity in your brain that initiates a chemical reaction in your body—your feelings. Some of these reactions are big and more readily noticeable, while others are quieter and harder to detect. Take your time here. Focus, and turn your attention to your body. This might feel a bit like meditating, but your goal isn't to feel calm on purpose or to only notice your breathing—it's to identify *whatever* you're feeling (and wherever you're feeling it), with no desire to change it. Much like not censoring your thoughts, you'll probably have to practice not ignoring or pushing aside your feelings. For this step, I like to do a gentle head-to-toe body scan, asking myself what my chest feels like, or my throat, or my fingers, or toes. Every feeling you have is unique, and some of them might be difficult to name right away. Do your best and remember that this isn't a test—nobody's grading you on the quality of your feelings or your vocabulary about them. Over time and with practice, this part of the process will get easier.

Decide if the feeling for that thought is good or bad

For this step, it's not essential to identify anything about your feeling more nuanced than a simple "good" or "bad." Knowing as we do that a good feeling will drive good actions—feeling motivated is what gets you into your exercise clothes and pushing the Play button on that workout video—while a bad feeling will drive you to waste time with avoidance activities like scrolling on your phone or mindlessly eating, or *in*actions like *not* drinking your water or *not* going to bed on time—then you don't need to get bogged down trying to parse out the difference between "irritated" or "annoyed." In the event that you simply can't decide whether a feeling is good or bad, skip that sentence and either come back to it later or let it go for now. Pro tip: Beating yourself up for not being good at this process feels *bad*, which means it's not helpful.

Write UNHELPFUL next to each thought that feels bad and HELPFUL next to the ones that feel good

I can't emphasize this enough—this is the part of this process that creates the most change! I'm going to explain these concepts in much further depth in chapters 2 and 4, but here's a quick rundown of how your brain makes changes. When your brain encounters something novel (like the recognition of an old thought being unhelpful), it pays more attention, just in case it needs to make an adaptation. Additionally, the act of writing the word *unhelpful* engages more of your brain than simply thinking the word, so this, too, is grabbing your brain's attention. And—sealing the deal—your feeling of relief or certainty or confidence toward the pronouncement of this thought being unhelpful aids in cementing this new concept in your brain. With just the simple act of writing one word, your incredible brain will do its job without any further intervention from you.

Let your brain do the rest of the work

For those of us who identify as control freaks—and I'm definitely talking about myself here—this step is the toughest one of all. I appreciate and applaud your desire to take charge of every aspect of this process, but the reason the Two-Step Tool works like magic is because it's what your brain is designed to do naturally, behind the scenes. By consciously labeling a specific thought as UNHELPFUL, you have tapped into one of your brain's superpowers: metacognition, meaning that you can think about your thoughts. In turn, meta-cognition triggers your brain's other superpower: neuroplasticity, meaning that you can think new things any time you want to. (We'll explore both concepts in greater detail in chapter 2.) In a nutshell: Your brain is capable of forming new thoughts and sweeping old ones away with simple instructions. Will the effect be immediate? For some thoughts, yes, but for others, you will need to be patient and persistent.

Using the Two-Step Tool for Other Goals

The Two-Step Tool can best be thought of as a compass, guiding you unerringly toward your goal. And throughout this book, we'll be using the Two-Step Tool to find your thoughts and decide if they're helpful with the specific goals of weight loss (chapters 2, 3, and 4), self-love (chapters 5 and 6), and acceptance of menopausal changes (chapters 7 and 8) in mind. But you can also use the Two-Step Tool to find self-awareness and create change *anywhere* in your life, with one key piece of information: Before you start writing in your journal, you want to be clear on your desired goal—either for the specific immediate situation or as a big picture.

Here's why: Let's say you're happily employed but have been dreaming of being an entrepreneur for as long as you can remember. When you sit down with your journal, you notice that you have lots of conflicting thoughts about whether you should stay at your job or strike out on your own. Without deciding on your desired outcome beforehand, you won't be able to tell if a thought like "I enjoy my job" is helpful or unhelpful, because it feels both good and bad, depending on which way you're listening to it.

If your stated goal is to remain with your company until retirement, then "I enjoy my job" feels very calm and comforting (a good feeling, so it's helpful for reaching your desired outcome of staying employed). But if your stated goal is to start your own business by the end of the year, then "I enjoy my job" feels like an anchor weighing you down (a bad feeling, which means it's unhelpful for fulfilling your be-your-own-boss dreams).

The same thought points in different directions, depending on where you want to go—so make sure you know where you want to go.

Are You a Thinker or a Feeler?

I'm loath to use the phrase, "There are two kinds of people in this world . . . ," but bear with me, because I'm about to lump you into one of two categories anyway: Thinkers or Feelers. In my experience as a life coach, I have learned that most women tend to identify—whether they know it or not—as one or the other. No matter which label seems to fit (or if both or neither of them seem to), you can successfully use the Two-Step Tool to get where you want to go.

A Thinker is a person who can readily hear the thoughts rolling around in her head and can capture them for examination because they present themselves—not every time, but more often than not—with some measure of clarity.

A Feeler is all about the body—a person who usually knows, seemingly intuitively and often without words, how she is feeling inside. This is not to say she doesn't resist or avoid her feelings like the rest of us, just that she's keenly aware of them in her body.

My whole life, I'd thought of myself as a Feeler—my emotions have always been written on my face, and I'm quick to cry or laugh or get angry. Additionally, as a fitness trainer and endurance athlete, I consider myself to be very in tune with my body's signals. And yet, when I started working on finding my thoughts and noticing the feelings they were creating for me, I learned to my great astonishment that I was quite disconnected from the physical component of my feelings. Instead, what I had always thought of as feelings were more like *reactions*.

Remember that your feelings drive your actions—that's their biological purpose—so when you are crying, or shouting, or throwing a plate across the room from anger, that's evidence that your feelings are working exactly the way they're meant to. But it's *not* evidence that you're fully processing (or even truly aware of) the feeling. I have been angry plenty of times without being even remotely conscious of the physiological sensations in my body.

I identify as a Thinker, and there's a chance—especially if you're a Feeler—that you'll notice my natural tendency to describe the first step of the Two-Step Tool as though it's much easier than the second step. Please don't take this personally or let it slow down your success. This is simply a product of the way my brain works best, and I encourage you to explore for yourself how you will be able to use this tool to your advantage.

The truth of it is that, biologically speaking, all of us are both Thinkers and Feelers—you have a working brain and functioning endocrine system (even if yours has challenges)—but you've likely learned in your lifetime to associate yourself more readily with either thinking or feeling, probably due to which one came more easily to you or was rewarded in your family of origin.

Let's Take This Show on the Road

Now that you know the basics of the Two-Step Tool, we're going to put it into action. I know you might think (or feel) that you're "not ready," but that's not a barrier to entry. At their core, both of the steps in the Two-Step Tool are simply *skills*, which means that if you don't currently know how to do them—and you don't, because nobody ever taught you this stuff in school!—you can learn to develop them, the same way you would learn to knit a scarf, or bake a cake, or fly a plane.

And by that, I mean you're going to practice.

In the following chapters, you're going to bust out your journal—or just a piece of scratch paper if that's what you have handy—and put pen to paper. At first it'll feel super awkward and useless and like you're not getting anywhere with it. That's completely normal, and why we're here working on this together. I'm going to show you my journaling pages—with the full transparency of my messy human brain and all of its unhelpful thoughts—and then we'll work on yours, too.

So grab your journal, and let's get started.

Everything We Learned in This Chapter

- Menopause has changed your body's processes, including the way you lose weight.

- Your brain leads the way in making changes to your body.

- The Two-Step Tool is simple, and really has only two steps: find your thoughts and decide if they're helpful.

- Your thoughts create your feelings, which then drive your actions, which is how you create results in your life.

- Simply thinking "good thoughts" isn't enough—those thoughts need to create good feelings in order to drive good actions.

- Far better than solving a problem, or helping you feel better, the Two-Step Tool will give you self-awareness.

- To find your thoughts, you'll ask yourself a question and write your responses in a journal.

- To decide if they're helpful, you'll ask yourself how you feel when you think that thought.

- You might come to this work with a natural affinity for thinking more or feeling more—both options are good, and you can learn the other as a skill.

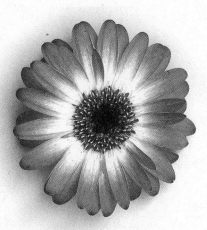

PART TWO

Losing Weight

CHAPTER 2

Estrogen, Calories, and the Lies We Tell Ourselves

~

Losing Weight During (or After) Menopause

Losing weight during and after the menopause transition gets a bad rap, with women all over the world declaring adamantly that "it can't be done" or "it's so much harder than it used to be." I'm here to tell you that it can be done, but it'll be different than you're used to. Weight loss has changed, just like your body's hormones. In fact, *because* of your body's hormones.

All these years, you thought estrogen was just giving you periods, but it turns out that it was working behind the scenes all along by

- helping your muscles recover from workouts,
- keeping your bones strong and dense,
- growing your hair (which is why it's now getting thinner and falling out and why lots of menopausal women don't shave their legs anymore),
- regulating your moods and physical stress response, and
- distributing the fat on your body in ways that made it easy to deliver and nourish babies.

With estrogen out of the picture, the things you used to do to lose weight simply won't work anymore. All those years of counting "calories in and calories out" or trying to "eat less and move more" are now more likely to cause you to gain weight instead of lose it.

Eating less = stress

When you think of stress, there's a good chance you're picturing "crunch time" with a challenging boss at your job or the relentless demands of being a caregiver for a loved one. You probably think that stress comes from being in a situation or circumstance that's outside your control, and I'm guessing that you know exactly what stress feels like in your body—a churning stomach, tightness in your chest and shoulders, a clenching in your jaw, and thoughts racing around in your head that don't ever seem calm.

And you've very likely heard that stress is bad for your health— that it causes weight gain (specifically, visceral fat storage in the belly and torso) that can lead to high blood pressure, heart disease, and other serious illnesses.

But do you know what surprising situation also creates stress— and the stress response of weight gain—in your body? Not eating enough. And do you know who undereats? Most menopausal women! Years of social conditioning have led us to believe that we have to eat less to lose weight, even if we're already eating very little. If I had to pick the most mind-blowing part of my weight-loss program it's this: You are probably not eating enough, and that might be causing you to *gain* weight.

This might be the strangest fact you've ever heard!

Everybody and their fitness trainer wants to tell us that we're eating too much and that in order to lose weight, we have to get into a caloric deficit because it takes 3,500 fewer calories a week to lose just one pound and blah, blah, blah. But nobody seems to mention what happens when you're already eating too little, so let me shed some light on this topic.

Let's say you're more or less my age (while writing this book, I was in my early fifties), you're an average height (5′4″ or 162 cm), you weigh somewhere around 160 pounds (73 kg), and you're exercising about an hour a day. Checking in with Google tells me that your basal metabolic rate—meaning the number of calories you burn by simply being alive and not doing anything other than existing (which is technically impossible, because as soon as you got out of bed this morning, you'd already started burning a bit more than that)—is just over 1,400 calories. Doing normal human things like having a job, eating food, enjoying a hobby, feeding your cat, or tending your garden means that you're likely burning at least 1,700 calories a day. When you add in an hour of exercise with an approximate burn of 300 to 400 calories, you should be eating about 2,100 calories a day just to maintain your weight.

But you're probably eating 1,200 calories or less, aren't you? Because your fitness app told you that was a great number, and we've all heard that number as the golden standard our whole lives. Even reading this right now, you might be thinking that eating in a caloric deficit of 900 calories a day really ought to make the weight just melt off like butter!

But that's not what menopausal bodies do.

Maybe that's how it seemed to work when you were younger—and that's a big *maybe*—but definitely not anymore. Now, your body thinks this underfueling is *stressful*, and we've already covered what happens when your body is stressed. It stores fat.

Estrogen Does What?

Here's a brief, *very* simplified rundown of what's going on biologically with menopause: Your body produces over seventy hormones (that we know of so far; there could be more) that are responsible for all your essential functions. For every hormone that makes something "start," there's another one that makes that thing "stop." For example, you have a hormone that signals to your brain when you're hungry ("start eating") and another one that sends you signs of being full ("stop eating").

Since puberty, estrogen has played a big part in regulating your periods. But it was also responsible for important jobs like regulating your body temperature and sleep cycle, protecting your memory and cognitive functions, stabilizing your moods, keeping your heart and bones healthy, and—the most important for our conversation here—attenuating the effects of cortisol, the so-called *stress hormone*.

Cortisol has a bad reputation in the popular media, but it serves several important purposes, including as an anti-inflammatory agent. Cortisol is the "start" hormone for quick energy when you need it (for example, in situations where your boss is demanding your time and effort, or you're taking care of somebody who needs you, or you've been undereating in an attempt to lose weight), because it raises your blood pressure and mobilizes sugar into your blood stream. Then it's estrogen's job to "stop" the blood sugar and blood pressure from rising and return your body to homeostasis (balance).

If you are chronically undereating in menopause, when you have little or no estrogen to counteract the constant surge of cortisol, your body stays in the "stressed" state of elevated blood pressure and unabated blood sugar, which then leads to fat storage. No wonder weight loss feels impossible at our age! Everything you've been taught your whole life about "eating less and moving more" to drop a few pounds is now completely wrong. Which means that everything I'm about to tell you is going to sound totally counterintuitive.

The 5-0 Method

Losing weight during menopause and beyond doesn't require you to give up the foods you love or mean you need to exercise all day. After a decade of working with many thousands of women online and dozens—including myself—in person, I've boiled the entire process down to doing just FIVE things every single day that'll make you say, "OH, I didn't know it could be this simple to lose weight at my age."

1. Eat the right number of calories, which probably isn't less than you've been eating.

2. Drink the right amount of water, which is half your body weight (in pounds) in (fluid) ounces of water.

3. Get the right amount of sleep, which means going to bed at the same time every night and getting up at the same time every morning without fretting about how much of that time was actual sleep.

4. Exercise moderately enough that you could put forth the exact same effort every single day for the rest of your life, which is almost definitely not more than you've been doing.

5. Manage your mind, which is using the Two-Step Tool (that we're going to discuss throughout this book!).

This Isn't Just a "Diet" for Your Body: It's a Lifestyle Change for Your Brain

The five things may sound familiar, and you might notice yourself feeling skeptical of their effectiveness. Because how many times have you committed to counting your calories, working out daily and upping your water intake, only to find yourself sliding back into old habits in just a few weeks or months?

Here's the secret: You are completely capable of changing your body by *doing* all the right things, but it won't "stick" until you learn how to *think* the right things that *feel* good to you. Which means—and I say this with so much love—that right now you are thinking the "wrong" things, unhelpful thoughts that are slowing you down and possibly even stopping you in your tracks instead of putting you on the speed train to success.

The 5-0 Method is so much more than that old "calories in, calories out" nonsense you've heard and tried a dozen times before, and it's definitely not a prescription for how to increase your willpower, which is an unreliable resource at best. This is diet freedom, radical self-trust, and beautiful self-awareness without judgment. Yes, even while you're counting calories.

The right number of calories

There are numerous calorie calculators on the internet, and every single one of them will give you a different number (which will be different from the number your calorie-counting app gave you), which feels super confusing. Online calculators will ask you about your current weight, height, age, and activity level because those are all important factors, but there are other variables—such as how much water you drink each day, how much sleep you get, and how much stress you have in your life—that can affect the calculation.

Rather than thinking of "the right number of calories" as being some fixed, objective number that you can calculate with 100 percent certainty that will always work, every time, for every woman, think of yourself as a beautiful experiment of one. Your body knows how much fuel it can take in and lose weight, and it will tell you very clearly (with lower numbers on the scale over the course of weeks and months) when you've found *your* right number. I'll show you how to calculate a number that's the perfect place to start, and I'll empower you to listen to your body and pay attention to your results over time.

Here's a very simple rule of thumb that can get you started: **Take your current weight (in pounds) and add a zero to the end.** For example, if you currently weigh 185 pounds, your daily calorie target is 1,850.

There are a few caveats, and this quick estimate will need some adjustments for certain heights, ages, and activity levels. If you are under 5′3″ (160 cm) tall, you'll want to reduce your intake by 20 calories per inch less, and over 5′9″ (175 cm) you'll add 20 calories per inch. For each year you are under fifty, you'll add 10 calories, and or each year over sixty-five, you'll subtract 10 calories. If you have a very sedentary job or hobbies, or are a person who prefers sitting, subtract 100 calories. And if you have an active job or hobbies or are a person you might describe as "fidgety" (like me), add 100 calories.

So, for example, if you are a forty-eight-year-old woman with a desk job and sitting hobbies who weighs 217 pounds and stands 5′1″ (155 cm) tall, your starting daily target will be 2,050 calories (2,170 from the rule of thumb, minus 40 for height adjustment, plus 20 for age adjustment, and minus 100 for activity level).

You have some *thoughts* about these numbers, don't you?

Why Is My Calorie Target So High, and Do I Really Have to Eat That Much?

You're likely asking yourself both these questions right about now, and in just a few pages you'll understand that they come from thoughts—opinions!—that aren't going to be helpful to get you where you want to go. But in the meantime, here's how your calorie target works for weight loss.

Your calorie target is "so high" because it already includes your exercise calories (meaning your anticipated calorie burn from exercise) in the calculation. Nearly every commercial weight-loss app on the market gives you a very low-calorie target and then, over the course of your moving day, adds in calories. For women over fifty, though, this "eat to exercise and exercise to eat" philosophy simply doesn't work. Your body, with its changing hormones, is not as simple as the calories in, calories out equation would suggest. More exercise is likely to cause you to gain rather than help you to lose weight.

As for whether or not you need to eat "that much," the short answer is yes, you'll want to hit your calorie target within +/-25 calories every day, consistently. The longer, more nuanced answer is that if you have been severely undereating—or overeating—for any length of time, you will want to approach your calorie target slowly, to give your body (and mind) time to adjust. I suggest starting where you are and adding (or subtracting, depending on which way you need to go) about 50 calories a day for the first few weeks, then another 50 per day for a few more weeks, and so on, until you get to your target.

What Is a Thought?

Your brain is the world's fastest and most powerful supercomputer, even though you sometimes walk into a room and don't know why you're there or you still occasionally need to use your fingers when counting. Every single minute of every single day, your brain is taking in thousands—probably millions, and maybe even hundreds of millions—of sights, sounds, smells, tastes, and textures, and then processing those perceptions into what you simply think of as the world. Reality.

It does this work faster than the blink of an eye through the use of comparison and categorization. Meaning that your brain perceives something (for example, the feel of the skin of your belly protruding over the waistband of your jeans) and then runs that thing through an internal checklist of everything it has ever perceived before to decide what it means and turn that perception into a *thought*.

Your brain goes through every single one of your past experiences—including but not limited to anything you've heard repeatedly from your mother or noticed even fleetingly from social media or television or your friends or billboard ads or magazines or that guy you met once when you were twenty-three but don't consciously remember—to compare and contrast with the current perception, and then it creates a thought to describe that perception: "I have a muffin top."

Along the path of those comparisons to your past perceptions, this current belly skin perception gets labeled into categories both broad and narrow, because it is similar to some of those old perceptions and dissimilar to others. For example, that muffin top might end up in the larger category of "uncomfortable," where you'd also find awkward social situations, hard plastic furniture, clothing that has even a trace of wool in it, and many, many other items, as well as the much more specific category of "things I don't like to notice about my body while I'm in the middle of a work meeting."

You've had many years of listening to people talk about muffin tops and seen countless ads and photos depicting such a thing. Even if you have consciously decried those representations as the hallmark of "diet culture," your brain is primed to perceive the skin of your belly over the waistband of your jeans as a muffin top, simply because you've been exposed to that idea repeatedly.

The first time you perceive something—an ad for a weight-loss product, for example, that promises to "melt your muffin top"—there are neurons in your brain that are making connections with one another along a pathway of sorts, which takes a lot of energy. Once your brain has spent this energy on comparing and categorizing, it will simply think that same thought again and again, because of your brain's biological drive toward efficiency or staying the same as much as possible to conserve energy.

You're Not as Rational as You Think You Are (and That's Okay!)

On the one hand, your brain is the most brilliant and powerful object on the planet, but on the other . . . well, your brain is just a piece of meat with electricity running through it! Sometimes what it does seems illogical, unless viewed through the lens of biology. Your brain, being part of a biological specimen (your body), has several biological imperatives, which you can think of as innate or even instinctual qualities that have helped us survive as a species for millennia.

Your body (and therefore your brain) wants to stay alive. This is not to say that you will automatically think thoughts like "Buckle your seatbelt" or "Wash your hands after handling raw meat," but rather that it will protect its resources to survive at all costs. What this means for you is that when your body is experiencing a drain on energy (exercising intensely or eating too few calories, for example) your brain's higher functions of logic, reasoning and rational decision making—the ones that take a lot of energy—will be deemed "extraneous" and shut down, or at least slowed, in a conservation effort to reserve fuel for more important functions like keeping your heart and lungs working effectively. Fun fact: Your body will also slow or shut down digestion under duress, because digesting your food takes a lot of energy. So, when you're undereating or overexercising, you could also be inadvertently slowing down your food motility and reducing your brain function!

Your body is primed to reproduce. Because of this, your brain and your thoughts are subject to all the hormones that regulate procreation. You have definitely noticed this in your lifetime. Do you remember being a teenager, when all you could think about was s-e-x? Or how you couldn't stop thinking about the donuts in the break room when you were about to start your period? Yep, that's your brain being *bio*logical (as opposed to *logical*).

Your body and brain want to stay the same as much as possible to conserve energy. This is because they take the long view of your life here on the planet and have allotted a certain amount of energy usage over your lifetime, like a frugal person on a fixed income who doesn't want to spend more than is absolutely necessary. Changing anything—your thoughts or your weight, for example— requires more energy than staying the same, so they'll only do so reluctantly.

Your body and brain are both capable of making adaptations when necessary. This is so that they can ultimately stay the same and conserve energy.

So, how does this show up for you on the daily? Your brain is largely running on autopilot, thinking the same thoughts over and over. And for the most part this is incredibly helpful —especially when you're doing something like walking, brushing your teeth, performing certain parts of your job, or even reading a book. Imagine if you had to decipher every letter of every word every single time you wanted to read a sentence. Or had to consciously think about lifting your foot and moving your leg forward and swinging your arm and holding your head upright just to get across the room. It would be exhausting and a huge drain on your energy stores, so much so that you'd likely need to be eating constantly (as many smaller-brained animals in the wild do).

Your Thoughts Aren't Facts, But They Think They Are

Everything we've covered so far—from the perceptions you've been forming your whole life to the biological mandates that run the show—means that your thoughts are pretty unreliable, frequently illogical, and biased in ways you might not consciously recognize. But this is all okay! It's just your brain being your brain. It doesn't mean you're not smart or capable or logical or truthful. It simply means that you're a human being with a human brain. It also means that you can stop believing everything your brain tells you, which is the best news in the world.

Let's go back to that thought, "I have a muffin top." As soon as your super powerful brain ran it through its complete database of other perceptions and landed on the conclusion of the "muffin top-ness" of your belly, it also decided that this thought is *true*. In fact, if you happened to notice that thought and questioned yourself about it, your brain would offer up all the evidence it had gathered while it was busy comparing and categorizing. Magazine articles, photos, ads, your friends complaining about their bodies and—as the info-mercials of my youth would say—*much, much more* would all confirm the veracity of the muffin top.

This is exactly how your brain is supposed to behave, by the way. It's called *confirmation bias*, and everybody's brain does it. Your brain likes to agree with itself and always thinks it's right, so it interprets all new information in ways that confirm everything else it has already thought. As a result, your thoughts are *always* going to contain biases and judgments that likely began forming before your memory even begins, and that all of your thoughts are going to sound true, as though they are facts—simply because your brain wants to agree with itself.

I know you know what a fact is, but I'm going to define it in order to contrast it with your thoughts (which *are not facts*). A fact is something that can be proven either true or false. For example, "I have green eyes" can be confirmed independently by other people, who would almost all agree (because you know there will be one person who has to say, "Well, they're sort of gray-green in some lights and blue-green in others . . .") that I do, indeed, have green eyes. Of course, if I actually had brown eyes, then my statement could be shown to be false, because the color of my eyes is a *fact*.

On the other hand, whether or not you have a muffin top is always going to be an opinion. And the way you know it's an opinion (which is a word that can be used interchangeably with "thought," because we don't think in facts) is that it *cannot* be proven either true or false.

Think about it this way: If you asked a hundred people to confirm your muffin top, some of them—women who are critical of their own bodies, if I had to guess—would say yes and prove the statement true, and some of them—maybe people who weigh more than you and are actually envious of how slim you seem to be in comparison to them—would say absolutely not, and prove it false. And some, of course, would be like, "What's a muffin top?" Ha! The point I'm making is this: There wouldn't be a consensus, because a muffin top is not a fact, it is an opinion. A *thought*.

How We Get (Unintentionally) Stuck in a RUT

Now, here's the real kicker: Your brain isn't going to offer up your illogical, irrational, and unhelpful thoughts in a straightforward way that you can hear and work through easily. No, the thoughts in your head—and sometimes even when you say them out loud—are going to feel like the truth, like something that you simply believe. But some of your thoughts are not good. In fact, they're Really Unhelpful.

RUT (Really Unhelpful Thoughts) is a clever play on words, but it's also a fun, simple visual for how your brain actually works. Thoughts that don't get challenged when they come in—and most of them don't—become automatic through repetition, and form something called a neural pathway.

When you think a brand-new thought, there are neurons in your brain that are making connections with one another along a "pathway," which takes a lot of energy. If there's no resistance to the thought, your brain will simply think it again and again, because of your brain's biological drive toward efficiency or staying the same as much as possible to conserve energy. Remember, nature is kind of lazy and wants to save energy now in case you need more later!

Then, as you think that same thought over and over, it will begin to require less energy and become more automatic, so it moves from the "front of your mind" where you can hear it to the "back of your mind," or subconscious, where it's still running on repeat, but you don't hear it consciously anymore. Over time, that thought forms a neural pathway in your brain in much the same way as walking the same route repeatedly through a meadow with high grass would eventually create a walking footpath.

As you get started with this work, you might feel overwhelmed with how many RUTs you find. Yes, you have Really Unhelpful Thoughts that are repeating themselves in your subconscious, but this is absolutely normal. I promise you aren't going to need to find and eradicate all of them to live an incredibly happy and productive life at your goal weight. The simple act of becoming aware of your thoughts (which is what you're doing when you use the Two-Step Tool) will begin to shift your life and your weight in ways that will feel like magic.

Thoughts About My Calorie Target
(What Honest Journaling Looks Like)

Since I don't have access to your journal to illustrate how to use the Two-Step Tool on your thoughts, I'm going to share mine to show you just how automatic our thoughts are. I am not currently trying to lose weight, but as soon as I asked my brain "What do I think about eating XXXX number of calories," my pen started flying! I had so many thoughts about that number, so many thoughts about my body and my weight and the efficacy of a program that contradicts advice I've heard my whole life—even though it's *my* advice! And I've used this program *myself* to lose weight effectively!

Your brain is not going to offer you facts, it's going to offer *opinions* that sound like facts. I was nodding my head while I was writing, totally agreeing with myself. It felt like I was writing a news article more than a journal page.

And even more than feeling *true*, my thoughts felt . . . yucky. Writing down your automatic thoughts is going to do what all thoughts do, which is to say that they're going to create feelings. And there's a better than decent chance that those feelings aren't good ones. (Remember, that's what this work is all about—we're actively finding our thoughts to see if they're helpful, and unhelpful thoughts create yucky feelings. So feeling kinda yucky while you're journaling and finding unhelpful thoughts is expected.)

While writing, I could feel my heart beating faster and my palms sweating. My stomach churned and my arms and legs felt "twitchy." I wanted to stop writing and get up and do something—*anything*—else. If this happens to you, don't worry. Stick with it as long as you can, even if it's just a few sentences. I've been practicing this for quite a while now, and I was able to find seventeen thoughts.

This is my raw, unfiltered, and unedited journal entry.

> **Journal Prompt: What do I think about
> eating XXXX calories?**

I can't eat that much.

I'll get so fat.

There's no way that will work.

What will I eat?

I'll be too full.

This won't work.

There's no way.

I can't do it.

I can't imagine that much food.

This is stupid.

I feel sick thinking about this.

I can't do it.

I don't want to eat that much.

This will never work.

Why do I even bother?

I'll never lose weight eating that much.

This is way too much.

Before we move on, I want to give you a couple of super quick "form tips" on how I write in my journal that allows me to get the most out of it.

- I keep my sentences very short, which is unlike my usual writing and thinking style. In "real life," my thoughts go on and on, with complex structure and vivid visual—and sometimes audio—accompaniment (because, yes, I talk to myself!). However, knowing that I am looking for specific information at the end of the session—is this thought helpful, yes or no?— means that I make adjustments to my writing in anticipation of that.

- I write one sentence (or even a sentence fragment) per line. Again, this is because I know that Step Two is coming. I want to leave room next to each sentence for the addendum that it's a thought, a space for identifying the feeling, and a remark about whether it's helpful or not.

- I don't edit the exact wording—however my thought presents itself in my head is the way it gets written down on the paper. When my brain offered me the word *fat*—even though I would never say it in public or to another person—that's what appeared in writing.

Are These Really Just Thoughts?

Next up, put the phrase "I think" in front of each of the sentences that follow, and take a moment with each one to absorb that it is a thought. You'll notice as you're doing this part that your brain is still thinking—it will offer you evidence of how the thought is true, tell you stories of other times in your life when this particular thing has happened before, and project worries into the future. Try very hard not to get distracted by this, but don't worry if you do, because it happens to all of us. You will always have more thoughts to examine—we think 60,000 thoughts a day!—so do your best to simply focus on the ones in front of you right now.

I *think* I can't eat that much.

I *think* I'll get so fat.

I *think* there's no way that will work.

I *think* I don't know what I'll eat. (Notice that I changed this from a question into a statement—we'll cover that in a minute.)

I *think* I'll be too full.

I *think* this won't work.

I *think* there's no way.

I *think* I can't do it.

I *think* I can't imagine that much food.

I *think* this is stupid.

I *think* I feel sick thinking about this.

I *think* I can't do it.

I *think* I don't want to eat that much.

I *think* this will never work.

I *think* I shouldn't even bother. (Again, changing a question into a statement.)

I *think* I'll never lose weight eating that much.

I *think* this is way too much.

Do you notice your mind already starting to shift? The simple act of putting the phrase "I think" in front of each sentence starts to allow your brain options, as though maybe—just maybe—these words aren't factual. Some of the sentences, though, still have that ring of "truthiness," which we'll tackle next when we decide whether the thoughts are helpful.

Questions Aren't Helpful Answers

When your brain offers you a question in response to your journal prompt, you will want to rephrase it as a statement in order to gain self-awareness. Remember how your brain always wants to answer a question? (*Wink.*) It sees questions as problems, and therefore automatically runs off in search of solutions. But when you're journaling, you're not looking to solve problems (or feel better)—you just want to see what your brain is thinking. As soon as you rephrase the question as a statement, your brain will be more capable of seeing it as a thought instead of a problem.

How Does This Thought Make Me Feel?

It's time to put each thought through a little test to see whether it's going to help you reach your weight-loss goal by asking yourself how you feel when you think it—because thoughts that create good feelings create good results, and thoughts that create bad feelings create bad results. (I'm repeating myself because it took a long time for me to truly understand this.) With the next step, we're looking to become aware of thoughts that feel bad.

Let's go through the list slowly, one by one, and ask, "How do I feel when I say . . . ?"

The answer you're looking for is as simple as "good" or "bad," though if you can identify a specific emotion, that's terrific, too. Just like when we added the phrase "I think" in front of each sentence, be aware that you are thinking more thoughts about these thoughts, and now about your feelings, too. This work takes a lot of focus! Don't be dismayed when it doesn't feel easy, or when you get sidetracked.

That's normal, and you'll get better with practice. Here's my journal entry again, with the feeling I noticed for each sentence.

I *think* I can't eat that much. [Bad/Horrified]
I *think* I'll get so fat. [Bad/True/Worried]
I *think* there's no way that will work. [Bad/Doubtful]
I *think* I don't know what I'll eat. [Bad/Worried]
I *think* I'll be too full. [Bad/Worried]
I *think* this won't work. [Bad/Doubtful]
I *think* there's no way. [Bad/Dismissive]
I *think* I can't do it. [Bad/Defeated]
I *think* I can't imagine that much food. [Bad/Unknown Specific feeling]
I *think* this is stupid. [Bad/True]
I *think* I feel sick thinking about this. [Bad/Horrified]
I *think* I can't do it. [Bad/Defeated]
I *think* I don't want to eat that much. [Bad/True]
I *think* this will never work. [Bad/Doubtful]
I *think* I shouldn't even bother. [Bad/Despondent]
I *think* I'll never lose weight eating that much. [Bad/True/Unknown Specific feeling]
I *think* this is way too much. [Bad/True/Dismissive]

Here are a few things to note about this part of the process.

- Remember that your feelings are created by your thoughts, not the thing you're thinking about. Here's what I mean: When you say the sentence, "I think there's no way that will work," and you identify that you feel doubtful, remember that the doubt isn't coming from the number of calories, or the program, or your body's ability to lose weight; it is simply a product of the thought. Thoughts create feelings.

- You don't need to be able to label the thought with a specific feeling for this work to be powerful. There were several sentences where I wasn't sure what I was feeling, but I could feel my lips start to purse and my shoulders tense. That's enough information to know that the feeling is bad.

- Some of your thoughts—maybe even all of them—still feel remarkably true, which seems more important than whether or not it's helpful. We all feel that way. So let's explore that feeling.

The nature of truth, and one of your superpowers

I'll just say it: **The truth is whatever you decide it is.** Of course there are facts in the world—you exist, gravity is a curvature of the space-time continuum, you have mass that can be measured by a specific instrument, and so on—but we so rarely think in facts that it's appropriate to just say we never do. Our thoughts are opinions, based on and in agreement with the perceptions of other things we've seen and heard in our lives, and as you discovered earlier in this chapter, that means your thoughts can be proven both true *and* false.

Your brain opts to believe that what you currently think (and have probably been thinking for years, efficiently and automatically) is true, because that's the path of least energy expenditure. But you are a human being with the power of metacognition: **You can think about your thoughts.** And this means you are not at the mercy of your automatic thoughts! Metacognition enables you to make permanent and lasting changes in your life. Rather than simply accept what your brain has offered you automatically, you can tap into your metacognition superpower and *decide* what you'd like to believe as truth.

"I don't want to lie to myself!" and your other superpower

I made that sound so quick and simple, didn't I? Decide what you want to believe and—*boom!*—your life is changed and everything is the way you want it to be. Yeah, *no*.

Your brain has safeguards in place to make sure that you won't change your mind quickly and easily (which would use extra energy), and you're noticing the most powerful one right now: discomfort.

You're thinking something new right now—maybe even a lot of "something news" about how to lose weight, how your brain works, the nature of truth, and the incredible power you have to change your mind and your life—and it feels exhilarating and terrible, all at the same time, doesn't it? Your stomach's a little squirmy? Maybe you're fighting the urge to pick up your phone and check your email or play a quick game of Homescapes? That's just your brain, wanting to conserve energy and stay the same. It's natural and expected, which still doesn't mean that it feels good!

In fact, if you're listening for it, you might notice that you have some chatter in your head right now about how you don't want to lie to yourself, so let me take this opportunity to assure you that you're not. You are not working to convince yourself that grass is blue and the sky is green. You are simply changing your mind about an opinion you currently hold, and you've definitely already done this in your lifetime.

When I was a kid, I used to hate eating rice. I don't know if it was because we ate instant rice, or maybe my mom wasn't a very good cook, or the fact that we only ate it in a dish my mother called the "Rice Special," which was rice with stewed tomatoes and ground hamburger meat (which still sounds gross to me). In any event, I made it well into my thirties thinking that I didn't like rice. And, as so often happens with opinions (which are just thoughts, after all) like this, I simply believed that it was true. A fact.

Until one day, I liked rice.

I have no recollection of the exact dish or the specific reason my opinion changed, but it absolutely did change. And now I love rice. It's one of my favorite foods and shows up in my dinner rotation several nights a week.

So, was I lying to myself when I thought I didn't like rice? Or am I lying to myself now that I do like rice?

Neither.

It's as simple as this: I had a thought that I believed was true, and now I have a different thought that I also believe is true. Neither are "true" in some universal sense, but both of them are/were true because I *decided*—in this case, subconsciously, but that's still your brain making a decision—that they are/were.

There's nothing about your weight, or the calories you need to eat, or your body, or exercise, or menopause, or your life that's different from my changing my mind about rice.

And in fact, being able to change your mind is one of your superpowers. Along with metacognition (the ability to think about your thoughts), you have neuroplasticity—meaning that your brain can re-form (bending like plastic) its own neural pathways. And you can be in charge of this rewiring process, by thinking new thoughts on purpose.

So, what can these two superpowers—metacognition and neuroplasticity—do for you? Together they form the basis of the Two-Step Tool, helping you find your thoughts and decide if they're helpful.

Fake It Till You Make It?

By and large, your brain (with its automatic thoughts) is doing just fine getting you through the day. The only time we really notice that it's not taking us where we want to go is when we're reaching for a goal like losing weight and need to make changes to our habits. You have enough willpower to override the automatic thoughts and make substantial changes in your life for very short amounts of time, but short-term changes (like a crash diet) don't get you to your long-term goals, and your automatic thoughts rarely change very much by themselves. This is where people love to offer you the advice to "Fake it till you make it," which sounds awesome—I mean, who doesn't love a good rhyming motto?—but it's an unreliable method at best.

Some proponents of the "Fake it till you make it" philosophy love to tout neuroplasticity as the reason faking it works, but simply repeating a new thought over and over does *not* change your mind. The missing element here? Emotional resonance, which means that a new thought has to feel good for it to "stick" and form a new neural pathway.

Lots of Your Thoughts Are Unhelpful, But Your Brain Doesn't Know It Yet

After taking a moment to identify the feeling each thought creates for you, go back over each item and label it as either HELPFUL or UNHELPFUL (remembering that the standard is that a good feeling equals a helpful thought and a bad feeling is an unhelpful thought).

I *think* I can't eat that much. [Bad/Horrified] UNHELPFUL

I *think* I'll get so fat. [Bad/True/Worried] UNHELPFUL

I *think* there's no way that will work. [Bad/Doubtful] UNHELPFUL

I *think* I don't know what I'll eat. [Bad/Worried] UNHELPFUL

I *think* I'll be too full. [Bad/Worried] UNHELPFUL

I *think* this won't work. [Bad/Doubtful] UNHELPFUL

I *think* there's no way. [Bad/Dismissive] UNHELPFUL

I *think* I can't do it. [Bad/Defeated] UNHELPFUL

I *think* I can't imagine that much food. [Bad/Unknown Specific feeling] UNHELPFUL

I *think* this is stupid. [Bad/True] UNHELPFUL

I *think* I feel sick thinking about this. [Bad/Horrified] UNHELPFUL

I *think* I can't do it. [Bad/Defeated] UNHELPFUL

I *think* I don't want to eat that much. [Bad/True] UNHELPFUL

I *think* this will never work. [Bad/Doubtful] UNHELPFUL

I *think* I shouldn't even bother. [Bad/Despondent] UNHELPFUL

I *think* I'll never lose weight eating that much. [Bad/True/ Unknown Specific feeling] UNHELPFUL

I *think* this is way too much. [Bad/True/Dismissive] UNHELPFUL

Now at this point you might be thinking, "Geez, Pahla, I've already been over this list of thoughts a couple of times; is this really necessary?" In a word, yes. Because this is how you tap into your neuroplasticity superpower.

Remember that your brain prioritizes staying alive above everything else (which is why it's always trying to conserve energy). And that means that—according to your brain—as long as a thought keeps you alive, it must be helpful. Truly, your brain doesn't care at all what you're thinking or how lousy it might feel, as long as it meets this incredibly low standard.

Your brain has put every thought you've ever had into this "helpful" category and now it's your job—with your metacognitive superpower—to change the labels and recategorize some of your thoughts.

I like to picture this like those old timey telephone operators who would work on a giant switchboard, plugging and unplugging the phone lines into specific slots to connect people. Imagine that you've been calling an "unhelpful" phone number for years and years, but as soon as the operator unplugs the line from that call and inserts it into a "helpful" slot, suddenly your call will go through to success. The Two-Step Tool doesn't have some "hidden Step Three," where you force yourself to think something positive and helpful. As we touched on in the box, "faking it till you make it"—simply repeating a positive-sounding mantra to yourself—doesn't change your mind all by itself.

Now, did you notice that all the thoughts I found about eating the right number of calories were unhelpful? That will happen to you, too. It's called "negativity bias," and we all have it. You are far more likely to have unhelpful automatic thoughts than helpful ones.

Scientists have found that all people have the tendency to notice bad news more than good, predict dire outcomes more often than happy ones, and attach more significance to (as well as dwell on later) negative stimuli over positive. Brain scan studies show a larger surge of activity in people looking at a negative image, versus a positive or neutral one, indicating that we *literally* think about something negative more than something positive. And even beyond paying more attention to something negative in the moment, scientists have shown that we hold on to that information longer and tend to give it greater credit when making decisions. While that negativity bias would have helped our distant ancestors survive harsh winters and predatory animals, these days it often makes us anxious and depressed.

One More Thing About Your Brain

Everything you've learned so far is all well and good on paper, but when you sit down with your journal and start looking at your own thoughts instead of mine, it's going to feel shocking how many terrible thoughts you have. I mean, holy moly, you are really good at beating yourself up. You say mean things to yourself all the time. It's hard to believe you've gotten this far in life with all the lousy things you've been thinking. UGH!

Ahem.

What I'm demonstrating here is a little something I like to call "thoughts about your thoughts," and it can be a real problem when you're new to journaling (until you notice it and use the Two-Step Tool on *those* thoughts and discover that they're unhelpful).

Let's circle back to two innate brain behaviors I threw out earlier in this chapter and stitch them together in a way that will resolve this issue: (1) problem solving as an evolutionary skill and (2) negativity bias. Your brain is really good at solving problems and therefore it is always looking for a problem. This would be awesome if it didn't also have a negativity bias that results in your thinking that *everything* is a problem. How does this show up on the daily for you (and everybody else in the world)? As judgment.

You are a Judgy McJudgerson. You judge the neighbors for how often they (don't) mow their lawn. You judge your spouse for opening even the simplest packages like a wolverine (which is a true story at my house—my husband doesn't believe in using scissors). You judge the clerk at the pharmacy for hanging on to that 1980s combover when being bald is actually on trend these days. You judge everyone and everything. And boy, oh, boy, do you judge yourself most of all. You even judge yourself for being so judgmental.

But here's the thing: you're supposed to be. This is, once again, biology dominating everything in its path and then running on auto-pilot. And your metacognition superpower is here to save the day, allowing you to *think about the thoughts that you have about your thoughts.*

Compassionate Observation

If the Two-Step Tool is the key that unlocks every door (and it is), then Compassionate Observation is the laser machine that cuts the keys. Or maybe it's even the locksmith who creates, uses, and deeply understands everything there is to know about keys and locks. The thing about thoughts is that we have a lot of them, and they're all just rattling around in our brain. We have a bit of agency over them when we write them down, but even while we're deciding if they're helpful or not, we are still somewhat *in* them, believing they're true and feeling the yucky feelings they create.

Compassionately observing your thoughts means taking a step *out* of your thoughts. It means noticing that they are sentences made of words—just ink on paper or pixels on a screen. It's taking yourself to a place that's free from judgment and open to the possibility of an alternate view.

Being a Compassionate Observer of your thoughts is not so much a state of mind as it is something you are doing—*observing*—from a specific feeling: *compassion.* You can do it any time you want by thinking a thought that creates a feeling of compassion for you. (Remember that your thoughts create your feelings and then your feelings drive your actions.)

For me, the easiest way to do this is to think of my thoughts as small children. I was a preschool teacher for a number of years, so it's easy for me to conjure up the vulnerability and irrationality of childhood. When my thoughts start throwing a proverbial tantrum about how *I'll never ever ever ever EVER be able to have what I want and it's just not fair and it's because everybody hates me and this time for real, I'm just giving up on my dreams*, it's very easy for me to picture myself getting down on one knee, looking my irrational brain in the eyes, and saying, "Tell me all about it, sweetie," while fully understanding that this is just how kids think and behave. They don't know better. And neither does your brain.

Another reliable trick for me is to think of my thoughts as small fluffy pets, like my dog and cats, who are essentially wild animals that have been socialized just enough to have a few manners and way too much to fend for themselves out in the world. Like very young children, they're helpless and occasionally opinionated but lack the verbal skills to communicate effectively. Truly, if you're picturing your thoughts as sweet, stubborn, immature, and a little bit dumb, you're on the right track.

The most surefire, effective way of compassionately observing my thoughts is to understand how and why my brain does what it does. This is why I've offered you so much cognitive and behavioral science so early in the book—it lays the groundwork for you to sit back and say, "Oh, of course I'm thinking XYZ because that's just what brains do."

Knowing that your brain is looking for negative thoughts, creating them on purpose, wanting to believe them as truths, and offering them to you repetitively as a matter of biological efficiency is the key to hearing and recognizing your thoughts for what they are: *just thoughts.*

Your Turn: Practice Finding Your Thoughts

If this is your first time journaling, there's a good chance you're feeling overwhelmed right now. I totally get it, and that's why we're taking a short break to practice this new skill, before trying to absorb anything more. Go grab a piece of paper and a writing instrument or open a new file on your computer.

Especially if you don't have a lot of journaling experience (or even if you do, because this method is likely very different from anything you've done before), your first attempt will probably not bear much fruit. This is to be expected! I encourage you to set your standards very low and then be super proud of yourself when you meet or exceed them.

Let's find *one thought*. Here's the question: What do I think about journaling?

1. Write down the very first thing that pops into your head, no matter if it seems related, or a "good thought," or whether or not it actually answers the question. *Boom!* There's your thought! (Remember that everything you think is a thought, so whatever appeared in your brain just now was a thought.)

2. Next, let's write "I think" in front of it. Do you recognize your thought as a thought? You might be aware that it's an opinion, but let's take this moment to really let it sink in that the sentence you just wrote down is a thought. It's optional. Your brain offered it to you, and you can decide for yourself if you want to believe it, even if you have lots of evidence that it's true.

    When you think this thought—just the one thought, not all the other ones that came before or after it—how do you feel? Good or bad? Or kinda good? Kinda bad? Kinda not much? If it's that last one, it's okay to stay here until you decide. There's no right or wrong answer.

3. If the feeling was good, write the word *helpful* next to your sentence, and if the feeling was bad, write the word *unhelpful*. Either way, take a moment to think about what this means. If it's your goal to learn how to journal and you found a thought that feels bad, then that sentence is unhelpful for your journaling

practice, and every time you think it, you'll be slowing down your progress. If you found a thought that feels good, hang on to it—that one's going to take you where you want to go!

Borrow This (Possibly) Helpful Thought

Even understanding that your unhelpful thoughts are *just thoughts* can still feel overwhelming when you first start this work, and that's why I'm offering you this (possibly) helpful thought. Think of it as a lifeline, so that when you feel like you're drowning in unhelpful thoughts about whether or not you can lose weight by eating at your calorie target, you can grab on to this one and keep your head above water. Why do I keep referring to it as (possibly) helpful? Because only you can know for sure—by applying the Two-Step Tool—if it's a helpful thought for you.

Here it is: *I am capable of thinking new things.*

Is it helpful?

As it happens, I love this thought, so it's incredibly helpful for me. When I think "I am capable" about anything—not just thinking new things—my shoulders instantly relax, my heart feels lighter, and my head feels clearer.

This thought creates a good feeling for me (calm confidence, which is one of my favorite feelings in the world), so it's a good, helpful thought.

But what about you?

Say the sentence to yourself and take a minute to notice what it feels like in your body. Don't worry if you don't know what the feeling is called, just decide if it feels good or bad.

If it's good, this is a helpful thought.

And if it's not, go ahead and label this one as UNHELPFUL and move on.

Everything We Learned in This Chapter

- Changing estrogen has changed weight loss, so "eating less and moving more" is now the problem instead of the solution.

- Your daily weight-loss tasks are eating the right number of calories, drinking the right amount of water, sleeping adequately, and exercising moderately—along with managing your mind about these tasks.

- The rule of thumb for your weight-loss calorie target is your current weight with a zero on the end.

- You have thoughts about that number!

- Most of the thoughts you think are automatic and driven by biology, which means they're usually illogical, stubborn, and resistant to change.

- Using the Two-Step Tool—which harnesses your superpowers of metacognition and neuroplasticity—can help you change your mind, think new thoughts, and get you where you want to go.

- The Two-Step Tool is (1) Find your thoughts, and (2) Decide if they're helpful, which means you'll write in your journal and then ask yourself how you feel.

- You're far more likely to have unhelpful thoughts than helpful ones, but that's okay, because you can decide to think helpful things on purpose.

- Compassionately observing your thoughts can get you out of them, which will help you determine whether they are helpful or unhelpful.

CHAPTER 3

Moving Less, Sleeping More, and Drinking Your Water

You might be wondering why, in a book about weight loss, it has taken this long to get to exercise. Or why I'm now grouping exercise with sleep and water as though it's a secondary activity. All five of the daily habits you build with the 5-0 Method are intrinsically intertwined and your success depends on being consistent with all five, but two of them—managing your mindset and eating the right number of calories—drive your weight-*loss* results. Exercise, sleep, and water, on the other hand, are more directly associated with weight *gain*, or at least hampering your losses. For menopausal women, exercising too much, sleeping too little, and/or not drinking enough water could be the reason you're reading this book.

Exercise and Weight Loss

Exercise is so, so, so good for you, but the truth of the matter is that it has very little to do with losing weight. So, first, let's dispel a few myths.

Exercise does not make you lose weight. Theoretically, if you are not currently exercising *at all* and eating your *exact* maintenance calories every day, you could lose weight by adding a nice, moderate 20-minute daily workout to your routine. In reality, however, this happens so rarely that I'll just go ahead and say it *never* goes this way. Most of us think that we need to "eat less and move more"—exercising for 60 minutes a day and slashing calories down to 1,200 or less—and end up throwing our energy balance into too large a deficit to be effective. Or we manage to do the opposite—offering ourselves high-calorie treats because we worked so hard today. And in either case, we're missing the beautiful complexity of our body and its fantastic systems. Weight loss does not depend on any one action in isolation but rather is achieved by a holistic approach that includes several aspects (like the five things we do with the 5-0 Method!).

Exercise doesn't burn fat. Yes, technically, exercise *can* burn fat, but your body more often uses other energy sources to fuel activity. When you take in energy (calories), your body can convert some of it into working fuel right away (your blood glucose, or blood sugar), but it will usually store some or most of the energy for later, in the forms of glycogen (which is a simple sugar that's stored in your liver and muscles and gets replenished constantly) or fat (which is stored either under the skin all over your body, or in the belly, and is designed to be stored there long-term). Stored fat requires more oxygen to convert into usable fuel, so your body is far more likely to tap into its blood glucose and glycogen stores for your workouts and the rest of your daily needs. There are theories that if you work out long enough or exercise in a fasted state that you can deplete your glycogen stores and "force" your body to burn fat, but even then your body has the option of catabolizing (breaking down) your muscles or other cells for energy. The bottom line is that your body will make fuel choices based on its own complex operating system that scientists don't fully understand, so your most reliable fat-burning bet is to eat in a slight caloric deficit consistently.

Exercising your abs doesn't burn belly fat, exercising your upper body doesn't reduce back fat or tighten up that loose skin under your arms, and exercising your legs won't give you a "thigh gap." If you take nothing else away from this book, know this: Your body is a little bit smarter than your brain and a lot smarter than the internet. If we had the ability, through natural means instead of surgical, to squeeze and shape our bodies into this year's "beauty standard" at will, we would lose some of our most important functions (not to mention our irreplaceable and unique beauty). You've been encouraged to pick apart your body for "flaws" since before you could understand what that meant, but your body is always taking a whole-body approach and making choices to keep you alive, healthy, and functional. Imagine if your body thought of itself in "parts" the way we do—your lungs wouldn't share oxygen with your feet, your heart would keep all the blood to itself, your legs would be running while your arms were staying still, and your brain wouldn't have dominion over any of it! Even though you might prefer to look a certain way, your body is much more clever than that. Storing fat in one particular part of your body is only a problem for aesthetics (with the notable exception of abdominal obesity being linked to heart disease), and sagging skin has no known dangerous side effects. Your body will store and use fat from specific areas due to its own unique combination of genetics and environmental factors, very few of which are under your direct control. Really, this was a long way of saying that you should exercise because it's good for your overall health and not because you're trying to force your body to look a certain way.

If you love to exercise, you're not going to want to hear this part

Not only does exercise not do what you think it does in terms of weight loss, but here in Menopauseland, it might even be to blame for your weight *gain*, as it was for me. Over the last fifteen-plus years,

I've run tens of thousands of miles and competed in well over a hundred races, including every distance from 5 km (3.1 miles) to 110 km (68 miles). I'm not an especially fast runner, but I have finished one race (at the 100 km distance, no less!) as the first-place female, and I have earned more than a handful of medals for running one of the three fastest times in my age group. On one very memorable occasion, I even qualified for the Boston Marathon—one of the only races in the world that you can't just sign up to run but rather must prove that you're capable of completing to a specific time standard. I run for fun. I run for sport. I run with my husband and kids for quality family time. I run when I'm happy, when I'm sad, or when I have something on my mind that I can't seem to work out any other way. I have run a marathon in a downpour with pelting rain and 25-mile-per-hour winds, and I have run an ultramarathon on a day that topped out over 100 degrees Fahrenheit. I love to run. I *really* love it, and I have spent the better part of the last two decades dedicating huge portions of my time, energy, and paycheck to this sport. To put it simply, running is my life. Or rather, running *was* my life. Until menopause told me to give it a rest—literally.

We learned in chapter 2 that estrogen has been helping us recover after hard workouts. The exact mechanism isn't clear, but for those of us who love to exercise, the repercussions definitely are, in the form of constant soreness, fatigue, risk of injury, general burnout, and unwanted fat storage. When estrogen was helping us recover efficiently, we could go, go, go to our heart's content. Sure, you needed to recover, but your timeline for that was speedy. For all but your highest-intensity days, you used to be back in the saddle (or your *exercise clothes*) the next day. And even after an exceptionally hard effort, you'd feel fine in a day or two. But now that estrogen has left the building, your workouts—at your beloved high intensity and long duration—could be doing you more harm than good.

I'm not a scientist or a doctor, so an exhaustive explanation of how your changing hormones affect your ability to exercise is well beyond the scope of this book. However, here's a rudimentary sketch of how your body reacts to exercise during and after menopause: While you are exercising, you are damaging your muscles with hundreds of tiny micro-tears. This is normal, and your body is fully equipped not just to "handle" the damage but also to repair itself so that it's stronger than it was before.

First, your immune system sends out inflammation to alert your body that there's been damage, and one of the first responders is the hormone cortisol. As we learned in the last chapter, cortisol—when it's working properly and in the right amounts—is really good for you, and acts as an anti-inflammatory while also raising blood sugar and blood pressure to keep your energy level up.

This is where the science gets murky. There are a few studies that show a correlation between lower estrogen levels and slower muscle recovery time, but the exact mechanism and interplay of hormones is both unclear and vastly understudied. What is known is that menopausal women take longer to recover from exercise, while also being at greater risk for insulin resistance (likely from the same hormonal exchange—cortisol raises blood sugar and without estrogen to help balance it, blood sugar remains high and eventually becomes resistant to insulin), and accelerated muscle wasting (again, possibly the result of reduced levels of estrogen not ameliorating elevated cortisol, which catabolizes muscle tissue to keep blood sugar high).

What happens next is a chronic stress response—one that you've likely noticed in your own body if you've continued to exercise at your premenopausal level of intensity—which includes the collection of fat in your belly and torso, mental fog, exhaustion, digestive problems, anxiety, and trouble sleeping. Yes, from exercising too much.

And even if you hate exercise, this still affects you

It's not just overexercise that brings on this chronic stress syndrome but the hormonal changes themselves, which means that your symptoms could be *worse* if you're not exercising at all. Unfortunately, the problems associated with a sedentary lifestyle include not just the belly fat, moodiness, concentration issues, and slow digestion issues I mentioned earlier, but additional serious risk factors like cardiovascular disease (even without obesity), joint problems, and poor immune system function.

The truth of the matter is that you can lose weight without exercising at all—because the main drivers of weight loss are (1) believing you can and (2) maintaining a slight caloric deficit over time—but that doesn't mean it's your best option. Your body is meant to move, it wants to move, and it functions at its best when you are moving regularly. The negative health impacts of lack of exercise are well studied and can be quite serious.

The Answer? Moderation

How much exercise is *just right* for weight loss during and after menopause? The amount that's just right for *you*—that is, "It depends." Moderation isn't a specific number of minutes, or a particular heart rate sustained for a fixed duration, or even a certain type of workout that you can do to guarantee weight-loss results. Exercising moderately is entirely unique to you, and it is based overall on your age, workout history, and current level of fitness or injury. On any given day, your workout may or may not be moderate for you because of how you've fueled recently, how much sleep you got last night (as well as the quality of that sleep), how hydrated you are, and your current level of mental stress. It's best to think of moderation not as a rigid or objective standard but rather as a sliding scale that could—and does—change from day to day.

How to find your moderate

My goal here is to give you guidance, as well as empower you to experiment for yourself and look for results over time, not only on the scale but also in the form of how energetic you feel for your other daily activities, your injuries (or, better yet, lack thereof), and your enthusiasm for exercise.

Here's a simple place to start: **Enjoy 23 minutes of exercise a day.**

Why such an odd number? Well, first of all, because exercising for 23 minutes a day, seven days a week meets (and technically exceeds) the standard 150 minutes of moderate activity per week recommended by the American Heart Association, the Centers for Disease Control and Prevention (CDC), and the World Health Organization, among others. Also, I have found that somewhere around 20 to 25 minutes is the sweet spot.

Of course, nothing about exercise or weight loss or your miraculous body is "one size fits all." As such, here are a few parameters to keep in mind.

- If you are currently injured and/or recovering from an injury, the only exercise you should be doing is your physical therapy. PT exercises are designed specifically to correct muscle imbalances and problematic movement patterns, so doing "regular exercise" on top of what's assigned to you could unintentionally be reinforcing the very patterns you're trying to change. Also, doing a workout in addition to physical therapy could be overexercise for you, which would negate the weight-loss results you're looking for. Remember that too much exercise leads to weight gain instead of loss.

- If you are currently exercising significantly more than this without injury, moodiness, or burnout, your body *might* be able to tolerate a longer duration. Reduce your workload to about 60 percent of what you're currently doing and pay close attention to your body's signals as well as to your weight-loss results.

- If you are currently not exercising at all, 23 minutes will likely be way too much exercise to start with, and could send your body directly into a chronic stress response. Start with no more than 5 minutes of intentional exercise, and gradually add another minute or two every few weeks.

You'll know that you are exercising moderately if you feel like you could do the *exact same workout* (duration, intensity, and size of weights, if you're using them) *every single day for the rest of your life*. If at any point in the workout, you feel like you're "really pushing it," or "feeling the burn," or "working hard," you're likely doing too much.

"I Don't Want to Lose All My Fitness Gains Just Because I'm Losing Weight!"

This is the worry I hear most from athletic menopausal women who love to exercise, but here's the cold, hard truth: You are *losing* muscle mass if you are exercising too much. Chronically elevated cortisol increases the protein breakdown in your muscles (muscle wasting), decreases the protein synthesis that would build new muscle tissue, and inhibits the release of the hormones responsible for muscle growth. This means that the best way to maintain or even increase your fitness is to exercise the right amount, which is probably *less* (either duration or intensity, if not both) than you're doing right now.

When cortisol isn't running rampant, your body will still happily build muscle (albeit more slowly than when you were younger, because you have to respect your menopausal recovery times), so this isn't the end of lifting heavy or running hard. You're still capable of performing athletically. It's simply the beginning of exercising *differently* for the fitness you cherish.

"It's Not Enough" and Other RUTs Your Brain Has to Offer You

I've just thrown a lot of information at you that's in direct opposition of everything you've ever heard about how exercise works and how to lose weight, so let's find and identify your Really Unhelpful Thoughts—or, more accurately, *my* RUTs—so you can move forward with the business of getting to your goal weight.

When I turned to my journal to capture my thoughts about exercising differently than I'm used to, and differently than I've heard I "have to" my whole life in order to lose weight, I found ten relevant thoughts. Below is an edited version of my journal entry (and I'll explain why I edited it in just a moment).

> **Journal Prompt: What do I think about exercising for 23 minutes a day to lose weight?**

I hate it!

It's not enough.

I can't lose weight without more cardio.

I'm not burning enough calories.

This will never work.

It can't possibly work.

This must be wrong.

I can't do it.

I have to do more.

I want to do more.

I could tell right away that these thoughts were likely to be unhelpful, because as I was writing I felt so much anger. Several times during the session, I found myself "going on a rant" and starting to write about the feeling of anger, and how betrayed I feel, and why this whole menopause thing sucks. And then I started to judge myself for having those thoughts!

There's a good chance you'll also find yourself going down a rabbit hole, and that's completely okay. It's part of the learning process, and it's good practice to notice when it's happening to you. But I reined myself in and came back to the topic at hand, and I encourage you to be on the lookout for "ranting" in your journal, too. That's because the outcome we're looking for with the Two-Step Tool is self-awareness—knowing what we're thinking—and that's most easily achieved with constraint to one topic.

Our brains naturally group ideas together (remember from chapter 2 that we are constantly categorizing our perceptions because we take in so many of them at a time), and there's no end to how many thoughts might be lumped into one "vent session." I visualize it like my brain going shopping at Target. I always walk in the door thinking, "I'm only going to buy shampoo," but suddenly remember that I've been thinking about replacing the throw pillows and might be running low on computer paper. This is my brain starting with the question, "What do I think about exercising for 23 minutes" and turning it into "What's everything that's ever gone wrong in my life, ever?"

Instead of giving your brain the credit card and letting it fill up the shopping cart at a store that has everything, do your best to remember why you're here (self-awareness) and how this work gets done (by following a formula).

These are thoughts, not facts

The next step of the formula is to recognize your thoughts as thoughts. Anecdotally, I've noticed that I have the hardest time with this part when the thoughts create feelings of anger for me. The more worked up I get, the more factual my thoughts seem. But they're still just thoughts, so let's write "I think" in front of each sentence as a reminder.

I think I hate it!

I think it's not enough.

I think I can't lose weight without more cardio.

I think I'm not burning enough calories.

I think this will never work.

I think it can't possibly work.

I think this must be wrong.

I think I can't do it.

I think I have to do more.

I think I want to do more.

How do these thoughts *feel*?

Also anecdotally, I notice that it's more difficult for me to parse the specific feeling for each sentence when the overall feeling from the journaling session is anger. For me, anger is a particularly unfocused energy, and I often find myself wanting to get up and walk it off. Remember, your feelings drive your actions, and this is proof! It may take some real effort on your part to stay focused on this task.

If—during the learning phase here at the beginning of your journaling practice—you find yourself unable to complete the entire Two-Step Tool process, don't worry. It's never too late to come back to your journal and continue where you left off. In fact, sometimes that's beneficial, as it offers you a distance between your thoughts, the feelings they create, and your self-awareness.

I think I hate it! [Bad/Angry]

I think it's not enough. [Bad/Worried]

I think I can't lose weight without more cardio. [Bad/Agitated]

I think I'm not burning enough calories. [Bad/Worried]

I think this will never work. [Bad/Resigned]

I think it can't possibly work. [Bad/Defiant]

I think this must be wrong. [Bad/Urgent]

I think I can't do it. [Bad/Defeated]

I think I have to do more. [Bad/Urgent]

I think I want to do more. [Bad/Longing]

Blurry Worries

Of the ten thoughts I found while journaling about doing twenty-three minutes of exercise, five are something that I call "blurry worries"—a specific type of unhelpful thought whose distinguishing characteristic is a lack of specificity. For example, thoughts that contain words or phrases such as "too much," "too little," "not enough," "more," "less," "not good enough," "too few," "enough," "too many," or some other nonspecific quantity.

Interestingly, the feelings these thoughts create are often "blurry," too. You'll likely have a sense of dread, or stress, or other unfocused yuckiness that you can't quite put your finger on. Particularly with the thoughts that create a feeling of urgency (see "This must be wrong," and "I have to do more" in my journal entry), you'll notice yourself wanting to just do *something,* even if you're not sure what.

On their surface, blurry worries can sound helpful, since they are usually directing you to do something that you think will get you where you want to go—doing "more" cardio, or eating "fewer"

> calories, for example. But because of their nonspecificity, they nearly always create feelings of unease, which puts them firmly in the unhelpful category.

Are these thoughts helpful or unhelpful?

Well, here we are, at the close of another great journaling session, with another list of thoughts that create bad feelings for us, so now it's time to let our brains know that all of these thoughts are unhelpful.

I think I hate it! [Bad/Angry] UNHELPFUL

I think it's not enough. [Bad/Worried] UNHELPFUL

I think I can't lose weight without more cardio. [Bad/Agitated] UNHELPFUL

I think I'm not burning enough calories. [Bad/Worried] UNHELPFUL

I think this will never work. [Bad/Resigned] UNHELPFUL

I think it can't possibly work. [Bad/Defiant] UNHELPFUL

I think this must be wrong. [Bad/Urgent] UNHELPFUL

I think I can't do it. [Bad/Defeated] UNHELPFUL

I think I have to do more. [Bad/Urgent] UNHELPFUL

I think I want to do more. [Bad/Longing] UNHELPFUL

Your Turn: Practicing the Two-Step Tool

Just like we did in chapter 2, we'll keep your journaling practice short and sweet, so you can get the hang of it without feeling too overwhelmed. You're just looking to find **one thought**, and here's the question: **What do I think about changing my habits?**

Write down the first thing that pops into your head, no matter what it is—there's your thought. Take a look at that thought for a moment to really connect with the notion that it's a thought, and then write "I think" in front of it.

Say the sentence to yourself, either out loud or in your head, and tune in to your body to see how it makes you feel. Is your heart beating faster than normal, or is your throat tight? Do your arms or legs feel jittery? If you can name the emotion that your thought created for you, that's great—but you can also simply identify if it feels good or bad.

If the feeling is good, write the word HELPFUL next to your thought, and if the feeling is bad, write the word UNHELPFUL. Again, take a moment to connect with why you're doing this—you have a goal that's going to require some habit changes, so if you're thinking something about changing habits that feels bad, you'll have trouble creating those changes. That thought is UNHELPFUL for reaching your goal.

Borrow This (Possibly) Helpful Thought

Remember that your automatic thoughts are far more likely to be unhelpful than helpful, and there's nothing inherently wrong with finding all unhelpful thoughts while you're journaling. The goal of journaling is to gain self-awareness, not solve your problems or feel better. Thankfully, part of self-awareness includes recognizing helpful thoughts, too, and the best way to do that is to occasionally brainstorm new helpful thoughts. Be sure to test them with the Two-Step Tool to make sure they create good feelings for you—and expose yourself to them intentionally.

Here's a (possibly) helpful thought about changing your workouts to lose weight: **I am doing the right amount of exercise for my goal.**

This thought feels particularly helpful for me for two reasons: First, it assures me that I'm doing the right thing (I love to follow rules—especially when I'm the one who creates them!), and second, it reminds me that I have a specific goal that I'm aiming for (and I love getting my goals). So the feeling I create for myself when I think "I am doing the right amount of exercise for my goal" is *calm certainty*.

Notice that this (possibly) helpful thought does not include the word *enough*. Rather than allowing your brain to think in "blurry" words, this thought contains a specificity that many people find reassuring. But does this sentence create a feeling of confidence for *you*? Or does it fill you with skepticism? Check in with your body and pay attention to your reaction. This is only a helpful thought if it *feels good to you*.

Sleep and Menopausal Weight Loss

How's your sleep now that you're here in Menopauseland? Pretty lousy? One of the most common complaints of women in menopause is the seemingly sudden onset of sleep disturbances. According to the National Sleep Foundation, approximately 61 percent of menopausal women have sleep problems, including hot flashes (night sweats), insomnia, and anxiety. If you're one of the women who experiences issues with sleep, you might not be thrilled to read that getting the right amount of sleep each night is one of the five main tenets of the 5-0 Method.

So let's start with the good news: You don't need to sleep perfectly to lose weight, and you're not doomed to stay at your current weight if getting your forty winks went by the wayside when you were in your forties. Adequate recovery and sleep are important for weight loss, but—like all the elements of the 5-0 Method—you're going to be empowered to figure out how much sleep is the right amount for *you* rather than trying to follow some generic advice.

Cortisol affects sleep, too

Hormones are so cool. The ways in which they interact with each other to control all of our essential body processes is endlessly amazing to me. Take cortisol, for example—the "start" hormone that raises your blood pressure and blood sugar to give you energy when your body is running low for one reason or another. As we've discussed, you might be low on energy because you're eating in too much of a caloric deficit, or you've just exercised intensely, so cortisol is dispatched to keep you moving through your day.

But cortisol has another important job that shows up for menopausal women: helping regulate your sleep–wake cycle. Your body regularly produces cortisol in a circadian rhythm—not just because of stress, but at times when your body naturally wants more energy—meaning that your cortisol levels are meant to be higher in the morning and lower in the evening.

You can imagine how disruptive it is for your sleep if you have chronically elevated cortisol, due to some combination of lower estrogen, undereating, and/or overexercising—or perhaps all three. If it's nighttime, but your body has morning-time levels of cortisol flowing through your veins, no wonder you can't fall or stay asleep. And then, come morning, when you're groggy from lack of sleep, what does your body do to try and get a little energy going? It spikes your cortisol even more. This is the very definition of a vicious cycle.

Making things even more "interesting" (note my sarcasm) from a weight-loss perspective is how a lack of sleep affects not just cortisol but other hormones that regulate processes like hunger, satiety, and blood sugar regulation. When your body isn't completing the normal recovery processes that occur with a full night's sleep, it seeks energy by increasing hunger signals and decreasing satiety—leading you to eat more and yet feel less full, while keeping your blood sugar high, which can lead to insulin resistance over time.

And then there are the night sweats

Speaking of vicious cycles, let's talk about the relationship between lack of sleep and thermoregulation (or the lack thereof that causes night sweats). The exact cause of hot flashes—which are called night sweats when you have them while sleeping—is unknown, but they are closely associated with the fluctuating hormones of menopause. For whatever reason, your body will suddenly have trouble regulating its temperature, and—*bam!*—your head and neck feel like they're on fire and your body is covered in sweat.

Night sweats are uncomfortable and cause wakefulness during regular sleep hours. In extreme cases, this nighttime thermoregulation problem results in insomnia. But do you know what happens from that lack of sleep? Your body temperature rises and has trouble stabilizing, which leads to more night sweats. Which leads to more lack of sleep. So, what's a menopausal girl to do?

The 5-0 Method Answer to Everything: Control What You Can and Let Your Body Take Care of the Rest

According to every article found in the first ten pages of my Google search, adult women (and men) need between seven and nine hours of sleep per night for optimum functioning. This appears to be an unimpeachable fact, and I'm not going to dispute it. I am, however, going to tell you to take this information the same way you took your calorie calculation from chapter 2 and the exercise recommendation from earlier in this chapter—as a point of reference in your ongoing experiment of one rather than an unbreakable law.

For a variety of reasons—not the least of which are the Really Unhelpful Thoughts we're going to explore in just a bit—you might not be getting seven to nine hours a night of quality sleep right now. Even though it might feel like the menopause cards are stacked against you, there are strategies you can employ to improve both your quantity and quality of sleep, and here's my favorite one: **Go to bed at the same time every night, get up at the same time every morning, and don't worry about how many of the hours in between were actual sleep.**

Do you feel skeptical about that advice? Fantastic—that means you have some Really Unhelpful Thoughts! (Why would this be "fantastic?" Well, the RUTs themselves aren't, but your burgeoning ability to recognize that you have them definitely is. Most of us start this mindset journey thinking we can simply force ourselves to think positively and get where we want to go through willpower. But now you're starting to realize that there are thought obstacles— RUTs—in your way, and the sooner you find them and label them as unhelpful, the faster you'll get to your goal. That's fantastic!)

Sleep RUTs

As it happens, I love to sleep. It's generally easy for me to make sleep a priority, and I have a solid sleep routine in place for both getting to bed and waking up. When I was preparing to journal about my approach to sleep, I thought to myself, "I don't think I'm going to have any unhelpful thoughts about sleep." And yet, when I thought that, I noticed a tiny little sensation of doubt.

How exciting! Maybe there would be RUTs to find, after all. So off I went to my journal, open and curious about what would come out of my pen.

> **Journal Prompt: What do I think about getting eight hours of sleep?**

That feels amazing.

I love to sleep.

Sleep is awesome.

Eight hours is good for me.

That's my regular schedule.

I'm not going to spend much time going over the Two-Step Tool process here, because you can see right away that these are all helpful thoughts.

I think that feels amazing. [Refreshed/Good] HELPFUL

I think I love to sleep. [Content/Good] HELPFUL

I think sleep is awesome. [Unspecified/Good] HELPFUL

I think eight hours is good for me. [Healthy/Good] HELPFUL

I think that's my regular schedule. [Content/Good] HELPFUL

How pleasantly surprising to find an entire handful of helpful thoughts! And don't let the speed with which I'm breezing over them here lead you to believe that I didn't take my time with them, because I did. Helpful automatic thoughts are a gift from your brain, and it will benefit you to spend the same amount of time—or more—with them as you do the unhelpful thoughts you find. Taking the time to write "I think" in front of each one helps to cement that this thought is an option, and you can choose it on purpose. Sleep doesn't feel amazing to you because of the nature of sleep, it feels amazing because you think it does. And intentionally labeling each thought as helpful will let your brain know that you'd like to continue thinking them as often as possible, thank you very much.

If I hadn't had that tiny inkling of doubt, these five sentences would have been the conclusion of this journaling session. But because I'd had that vague feeling of doubt, I decided to come at this from another angle.

The first question isn't always the right question, and it's okay to ask more

Your journaling practice will take on its own personality over time, and it's one of my goals with this book to show you that this journaling journey is *yours*—even though I'm offering you very specific, detailed, and prescriptive advice on exactly how to journal. You own it. You are creating it. It is about you, and for you. Have fun with it, play with it, and be curious about it. Know that there's always another way to find what you're looking for when what you're looking for is self-awareness.

There's always another question to ask yourself, and there's no such thing as a bad question. Sometimes, you'll find that a question elicits painful responses that feel so true you struggle to gain any agency over them, or you may ask a question that your brain meets with a stone wall of "I don't know," or—like the previous Journal Prompt example—you might not find the unhelpful thoughts that are slowing you down from getting to your goal. Any of these situations may feel like a "bad journaling session," but I encourage you to recognize that as an unhelpful thought. The best journaling session is the one you get done.

In this case, the session that got it done needed two questions, including this next one, where I found the unhelpful thoughts that had been lurking in the background. Now that you're getting more familiar with the Two-Step Tool, I'll move through the process with shorter explanations. But feel free to reference the last section of chapter 1 if needed.

> **Journal Prompt: What do I think about sleeping eight hours a night?**

I can't stay asleep.

I have to wake up with Blossom. (Blossom is my elderly, semi-incontinent dog.)

I get too hot.

I can't.

I always have to pee.

Sometimes it's hard.

I never sleep all night.

I'm having so many night sweats.

I'll never sleep through the night again.

Pay dirt! I found nine relevant thoughts, and while I was writing, I found myself nodding and agreeing with myself. "Yep. Yep. This is absolutely true. OMG, I *am* having so many night sweats lately!" So, I made sure to go over each line very carefully while I added "I think" in front of each one, and I really took the time to recognize these thoughts as thoughts. I reminded myself that they are opinions. They are sentences that are neither true nor false but solely my brain's interpretation of its perceptions. These are stories I'm telling myself, and that means they are optional.

I think I can't stay asleep.

I think I have to wake up with Blossom.

I think I get too hot.

I think I can't.

I think I always have to pee.

I think sometimes it's hard.

I think I never sleep all night.

I think I'm having so many night sweats.

I think I'll never sleep through the night again.

After I sat with each sentence and recognized it as a thought (instead of a fact), I was able to tune in and notice the feelings they created in my body.

I think I can't stay asleep. [Bad/Defeated]

I think I have to wake up with Blossom. [Bad/Irritated]

I think I get too hot. [Bad/Frustrated]

I think I can't. [Bad/Resigned]

I think I always have to pee. [Bad/Put-Upon]

I think sometimes it's hard. [Bad/Whiny]

I think I never sleep all night. [Bad/Indignant]

I think I'm having so many night sweats. [Bad/Frustrated]

I think I'll never sleep through the night again. [Bad/Doomed]

And finally, I intentionally labeled each thought that created a bad feeling as UNHELPFUL, and I reminded myself again that—because they are just opinions and interpretations—these thoughts are neither true nor factual.

I think I can't stay asleep. [Bad/Defeated] UNHELPFUL

I think I have to wake up with Blossom. [Bad/Irritated] UNHELPFUL

I think I get too hot. [Bad/Frustrated] UNHELPFUL

I think I can't. [Bad/Resigned] UNHELPFUL

I think I always have to pee. [Bad/Put-Upon] UNHELPFUL

I think sometimes it's hard. [Bad/Whiny] UNHELPFUL

I think I never sleep all night. [Bad/Indignant] UNHELPFUL

I think I'm having so many night sweats. [Bad/Frustrated]
UNHELPFUL

I think I'll never sleep through the night again. [Bad/Doomed]
UNHELPFUL

All-or-Nothing Thinking

One of the skills you'll develop as you practice journaling is spotting when your brain offers you a particular kind of unhelpful thought, like the Blurry Worries. (Did you spot the Blurry Worries in this latest example? No problem if you didn't—this isn't a test, and I'm going to point them out to you. There were two: "I get *too* hot," and "I'm having *so many* night sweats.")

All-or-Nothing Thinking is a specific unhelpful thought characterized by extremist language—words such as *all, always, forever, nothing,* or *never.* Of the nine thoughts I found with this question, three of them included All-or-Nothing Thinking: "I always have to pee," "I never sleep all night," and "I'll never sleep through the night again." Once I saw the telltale words, I could recognize immediately that those thoughts were unhelpful (though I still identified the feelings they created, because that's good practice).

Cognitive behavioral therapists refer to categories of unhelpful thoughts like these as *cognitive distortions* or *thought errors.* For my own amusement—and because I'm a huge fan of using mnemonic devices to remember information—I have come up with silly or repetitive names for some of the most common thought errors. I call this particular thought error ANTs (All or Nothing Thinking). As in, "Oh, here come the ANTs, trying to ruin the picnic."

Language matters

The difference in wording between "What do I think about getting eight hours of sleep?" versus "What do I think about sleeping eight hours a night?" is so subtle it's almost unbelievable how different my responses were, right? Why would one of those questions produce all helpful thoughts and the other garner nothing but unhelpful thoughts? Brains are wonderful and mysterious beings, that's why, and they respond to specific nuances of language because of your unique life experiences.

Here's my theory about why these two questions landed the way they did: To me, the first one (with the helpful responses) sounded like I was asking about the *theory* of *a person* sleeping eight hours, whereas the second one (with the unhelpful answers) seemed very much a question about whether or not I, personally, was capable of sleeping for that length of time. Your brain will have idiosyncrasies like this, too, so empower yourself to brainstorm your own questions if you find that the Journal Prompts I provide don't resonate with you.

Your Turn: Finding Your Thoughts about Your Thoughts

Grab a piece of paper—the one you used for the other journal prompts earlier is fine—and a writing implement, and let's find **one thought** with this question: **What do I think about finding my thoughts?**

It might be meta, but go ahead and write down your thought—even if it feels like a fact right now—about finding your thoughts. And then write "I think" in front of it while allowing your brain to absorb the idea that this sentence isn't factual information.

How does your thought make you feel? Remember to check in with your body instead of just listening to more thoughts about your thoughts. If you feel good, write HELPFUL next to your thought. If you feel bad, write UNHELPFUL and take a moment to process what this means: The thought you're having about finding your thoughts isn't going to help you find your thoughts.

Borrow This (Possibly) Helpful Thought

When it comes to menopausal women and helpful thoughts about sleep, I often find that you don't need to aim for something that feels ecstatic, or amazing, or even "really good." In fact, what might be the most helpful for you is to use relatively neutral language that merely acknowledges the fact that you sleep. As such, my recommendation for a (possibly) helpful thought is this: **I have a sleep schedule.**

Because you *do*. Your current sleep schedule might be erratic and plagued with frustrating wakefulness, but it's still a schedule. The way this sentence dances lightly between being technically true (but maybe only through omission) and ever-so-slightly aspirational is exactly what you're looking for in a helpful thought. Well, that and the fact that it produces a good feeling in you, of course.

For me, the thought "I have a sleep schedule" feels calm and grounding, like a decision I've already made and don't have to worry about anymore. It's a pleasant reminder that I am in control of my timing, and blissfully ignores that I'm not in control of the finer details of how much or how well I sleep within that schedule.

Take a moment to notice how this thought feels to you. Does it evoke disbelief? Certainty? Or something in between? If this thought feels good to you, it's helpful, and if it feels bad, feel free to label it as UNHELPFUL and move on.

Drinking Water to Lose Weight

Every single cell in your body needs water to perform its complex and miraculous processes. So why do so many women think of staying hydrated as a chore? Because we have Really Unhelpful Thoughts about drinking water, of course! But before we explore those RUTs, let's explore how and why drinking an adequate amount of water is essential for your weight-loss goals.

Your body doesn't store hydration the way it stores energy—you can live for weeks without eating, but you will die in about three days without drinking. Further, your amazing body can adapt and still thrive in a wide variety of circumstances—weather that's very hot or very cold, poor or sporadic nutrition, changes in elevation and humidity, and by growing or depleting muscle mass in response to activity level. But the one and only thing that your body *cannot* adapt to is dehydration.

Instead of making adaptations in the face of water shortage, your body will simply shut down processes that it considers extraneous, such as higher-level cognitive functioning (making decisions) and food motility (digestion). Yes, what I'm saying here is that both your brain and your body get constipated when you're not drinking enough water.

Water doesn't help you lose weight by "filling you up" or suppressing your appetite (two very common myths that I hear daily and vehemently dispute whenever I can). But it does assist in your weight-loss journey by allowing your body to operate its fueling systems (your metabolism) at peak efficiency—meaning that you are digesting food quickly, moving fuel and nutrients around effectively to the body parts that need them, and regularly producing appropriate waste.

In addition to helping you lose weight, drinking adequate water will soften your hair, moisten your skin and lips enough to go without lotions and balms, and prevent you from getting that dizzy feeling when you stand up quickly. Did you know that was from dehydration? Drink your water and feel the difference.

How much water is enough?

There's a super simple formula to calculate an adequate amount of hydration for your body: **Drink half your body weight (in pounds) in fluid ounces of water.**

Uhhhhh . . . Pahla, that's a LOT of water!

I know this number might feel shocking when you first hear it, because we've all been told our whole lives that 8 glasses a day is the standard we're aiming for. And this is fabulous if you weigh 128 pounds, because then you don't need to change a thing. But the rest of us will want to make adjustments in order to drink the right amount of water for our particular body's needs.

Here are a few points to keep in mind, as you aim to meet this daily water target.

- If you have a medical condition that requires you to limit your water, you should adhere to your doctor's plan.

- If you take in too much at once, you'll just pee it all out. Think of flooding a plant that hasn't been watered in weeks—the soil can't absorb all the water at once, so it will leak to the bottom of the container and get absorbed slowly over time. Unfortunately, you don't have a vessel to reabsorb your overfilled kidneys, so drink slowly over the course of your day. I suggest drinking water with (or at least near) your meals, which will give the water something to "soak into," and also promote better digestion of your food.

- Watery foods (such as soups, grapes, or watermelon) and other fluids (such as coffee, tea, soda, or juice) do contribute to hydrating your body and can "count" toward your daily target. For best results, though, I suggest that you meet your water target with only water at first, and pay attention to the results you get over time. Some women get fabulous weight-loss results by counting everything, and some—me, for example—need to be very precise with our water.

- If you're currently drinking much less than your target, your body will need time to adjust (and the additional water will likely show up on the scale as a gain in the first few days or even weeks). Add 8 ounces to your daily regimen every two to three weeks until you are meeting your target. You might still need frequent bathroom breaks when you get started, but adding slowly over time can reduce this inconvenience.

Water RUTs

I vividly remember my New Year's Resolutions going into 1981, when I was eleven years old—at the top of the list was "Drink more water." (Other items included, "Be nicer to people," and "Don't eat so many cookies.")

I don't know how much water I was drinking at the time, or where I'd heard that I needed to drink "more," but I do know that I'd already had many years of Really Unhelpful Thoughts about my (supposed) inability to drink water, and I was facing many more in front of me. Within the month, I stopped trying to drink more water and gave up on myself as a lost cause—thanks to my efficient, automatic thoughts.

In fact, these RUTs about drinking water were so pervasive and long-lasting that I only had to go back a few years in my old journals to find an entry about finally meeting my intake. Here are some excerpts from my journal at the time that you might find useful as you think about upping your water intake.

> **Journal Prompt: What do I think about drinking XX ounces of water every day?**

I'll never be able to drink that much.

I won't stick with it.

I'll have to pee all the time.

I don't like how water tastes.

It's too hard to drink that much.

I'll feel so sloshy.

That's a lot of water.

The problem with true opinions

When you are journaling, you'll find yourself occasionally butting up against something I call *true opinions*, which are thoughts that you can clearly recognize as being opinions—"I don't like the taste of water" is the one I found here—that you don't know what to do with. I mean, you can't *mindset* your way out of not liking water, right?

Well, technically, yes, you can. But more important, you don't have to. And before I explain why that is, let me offer you a gentle reminder that we come to our journal only for self-awareness rather than trying to solve a problem or because we want to feel better.

When you come across a true opinion that is clearly in opposition to meeting your goal, your amazingly powerful and speedy brain takes a couple of steps, which then spirals into a loop that you likely don't consciously hear but that has the power to stop you in your journaling tracks. First, your brain identified the thought "I don't like the taste of water" as a problem—you have to drink water to lose weight, but you don't like water, so you won't be able to lose weight. That's a problem. Then, your brain immediately went to work finding a solution to that problem—you'll have to learn how to like water.

But you don't like water.

Your brain will go around and around, trying to solve this unsolvable problem in an effort to feel better, because not being able to solve a problem—remember that it's your brain's main function to look for and solve problems—feels terrible. In fact, it's another problem! So this is why we come to our journal with only the intention of finding self-awareness: There are no problems, there's just information.

Knowing that your brain operates under the assumption that everything is a potential problem and that it wants to solve any problem it finds means that while you're journaling, you'll want to be on the lookout for true opinions. Thankfully, you handle them the same way you manage all of your "regular" thoughts—by putting them through the Two-Step Tool and recognizing that they're thoughts.

THESE SENTENCES ARE THOUGHTS...

I think I'll never be able to drink that much.

I think I won't stick with it.

I think I'll have to pee all the time.

I think I don't like how water tastes.

I think it's too hard to drink that much.

I think I'll feel so sloshy.

I think that's a lot of water.

...THAT CREATE FEELINGS

After you give yourself a minute to really take in the idea that these (very true-sounding!) statements are thoughts, it's time to identify your feelings.

I think I'll never be able to drink that much. [Bad/Dismissive]

I think I won't stick with it. [Bad/True/Ashamed]

I think I'll have to pee all the time. [Bad/Worried]

I think I don't like how water tastes. [Bad/Disgusted]

I think it's too hard to drink that much. [Bad/True/Indignant]

I think I'll feel so sloshy. [Bad/Worried]

I think that's a lot of water. [Bad/True/Rejecting]

... WHICH ARE EITHER HELPFUL OR UNHELPFUL

And then, the last step, we'll finish up by labeling the thoughts as UNHELPFUL, and letting the consequences of that decision sink in. These thoughts are not going to help you get to your water-drinking target or your ultimate weight-loss goal.

I think I'll never be able to drink that much. [Bad/Dismissive]
UNHELPFUL

I think I won't stick with it. [Bad/True/Ashamed] UNHELPFUL

I think I'll have to pee all the time. [Bad/Worried] UNHELPFUL

I think I don't like how water tastes. [Bad/Disgusted] UNHELPFUL

I think it's too hard to drink that much. [Bad/True/Indignant]
UNHELPFUL

I think I'll feel so sloshy. [Bad/Worried] UNHELPFUL

I think that's a lot of water. [Bad/True/Rejecting] UNHELPFUL

Predicting the Future

There's another category of specifically unhelpful thoughts that I like to call Predicting the Future . . . because they are thoughts that predict something (usually a terrible outcome) that could possibly happen in the future. You can spot these Predicting the Future thoughts by looking for the words *will* or *won't*. Your brain will offer you these thoughts, not as guesses or possible suppositions, but as though the results are certain—exactly the way I just did in this sentence.

The ability to quickly sort through everything you've ever perceived in the past and predict what's coming next is quite helpful when it comes to things like defensive driving, performing life-saving surgery, or even having a conversation with a friend. But when it comes to getting your goal, this skill can produce Really Unhelpful Thoughts.

The truth of it is, you have no idea what's going to happen in the future. You might wake up and pee seven times from drinking an adequate amount of water, or you might not. Recognize that this is an unhelpful thought and don't let it stop you from drinking the water.

Your Turn: Find Your Thoughts about Doing New Things

Here we are with more super quick journaling practice—soon you're going to be a pro and won't need me anymore! Let's find **one thought** in answer to this question: **What do I think about doing new things?**

Write down the first thing you heard in your head in response, and let it sink in that this is a *thought*. Write "I think" in front of it and read it to yourself again. How do you feel when you think that thought—good or bad?

If the thought feels good, write HELPFUL next to it and make a mental note to think it as often as possible. If, on the other hand, the thought feels bad, write UNHELPFUL next to it and allow your brain to gently remove it from the thought rotation at its own pace.

Borrow This (Possibly) Helpful Thought

You're about to learn something embarrassing about me. I love some inappropriate humor. I would blame it on being the mother of two boys, but the truth is that I've loved a good bathroom joke since long before my kids came around. I mention this because my own helpful thought around hydration (that could possibly be helpful for you) is this: **Drinking water gets me everywhere I want to go.**

It makes me chuckle every time I think it, and that's how I know it's a helpful thought—I feel good. It's funny, it's scientifically truthful, it feels believable, and it doesn't sound nagging, like the (un) helpful thoughts we usually tell ourselves about how "I have to drink water because it's good for me" or "I need to drink enough water or I'll never lose this weight."

How does this thought feel to *you*? If it creates a good feeling, it's helpful, but if it feels bad, it can get chucked into the "unhelpful" bin right away.

Everything We Learned in This Chapter

- Exercise is not the main driver of weight loss, and it could even be the cause of weight gain for menopausal women.

- Without estrogen to attenuate the presence of cortisol, your body can develop a chronic stress response to a level of exercise that used to be fine before menopause.

- Instead of exercising "more" to lose weight, you want to exercise the right—moderate—amount, which allows your body to recover properly.

- Your changing hormones can also change how well you sleep, due to menopausal symptoms such as insomnia and night sweats.

- Having a consistent sleep schedule helps with weight loss, even if your quality of sleep is different from what it was before menopause.

- Drinking an adequate amount of water is essential for all of your body's processes, not to mention that it helps you with weight loss.

- Your brain has specific categories of unhelpful thoughts—thought errors such as Blurry Worries, All-or Nothing Thinking, and Predicting the Future—that you can recognize and intentionally recategorize.

- The Two-Step Tool is designed for self-awareness, not as a solution to a problem or to help you feel better.

CHAPTER 4

Scale Thoughts

How Much Do You Want to Weigh?

You're reading a book about weight loss, and you probably think a lot about how desperately you want to lose weight, but do you know how much you want to weigh? Yes, I'm asking if you have a *number* in mind. I'm going to venture a guess that you have *sort of* an idea of the weight you'd like to be, but that it skitters around in your mind, like, "I want to lose fifty pounds, but I'd be okay if I lost forty. Or thirty . . . and honestly, I'd be happy if I could just get rid of ten pounds." Or, if you can get hold of a firm, clear number, you're filled with doubts about whether that weight is reasonable, or if you're capable of getting to it, or if it's even a good idea because if you get there you probably won't be able to maintain it, or what if people think you're too thin? Having a specific target in mind is crucial, though, because your brain can't focus on (or arrive at) a destination like "not fat" or "maybe if I lose ten or twenty pounds."

Imagine if you wanted to take a vacation but didn't choose where you'd like to go. You wouldn't be able to buy plane tickets, you wouldn't be able to book a hotel reservation, you wouldn't know what to pack or when to take time off from work. You'd be stuck before you even got going! But once you decide that you'd like to visit New York City on December 31 so that you can watch the ball drop in Times Square—well, now you're talking. You know you'll need to book far in advance of such a big event to secure plane tickets at reasonable prices, you can scout out a hotel close enough to walk to and from the festivities, and you'll be sure to bring your warmest boots and gloves. When you know exactly where you're going, you can plan for the trip and anticipate it with excitement.

Remember that your feelings drive all your actions, so if you are feeling wishy-washy or confused or unclear, you will not be able to move forward with purpose toward your goal. When you feel certain or excited—because you know exactly where you're going and what it's going to feel like when you get there—your brain will keep pointing you in the right direction.

How to Decide on Your Goal Weight

I used to be an "overthinker." Maybe you can relate? Every decision I made, even something as simple as what to have for dinner, required a pages-long list of pros and cons. I had endless debates with myself about the smallest, most mundane decisions and drove myself bonkers by waffling. I think most people make decisions like this, even if they don't call themselves overthinkers. Many of us tend to believe that all the thinking should come before the decision, as though by weighing the possibilities, we can somehow ensure the outcome we desire. But now that I manage my own mind regularly (and help you manage yours for a living), I completely disagree. The fact is, you can't predict the future (remember from chapter 3 that Predicting the Future thoughts are usually unhelpful), but you can shape it by setting yourself a goal. Rather than trying to analyze things that you *cannot know*, simply decide the direction in which you want to be heading, then wait until you have some data to see if you're getting there.

Nowadays, I consider myself decisive about most things, and on the rare occasions when I find myself dithering, I know exactly how to get out of it. Here is my super simple formula for making any decision (including the one about what you want to weigh).

1. **Make the decision.** First of all, I know it's funny that step one of making decisions is to make the decision! But it is actually that simple. Remember, **the truth is what you decide it is,** and you are going to have automatic thoughts no matter what. So just decide. Pick something out of thin air if you want to.

2. **Commit to finding your thoughts about the decision.** You are going to have thoughts. You always do, you always will, and they will nearly always be automatic (and usually unhelpful) until you find them and decide if they're helpful. Rather than trying to do all your thinking first, commit to paying attention to your thinking *after* the decision is made, so you can move forward in the direction you want to go.

3. **Set a time in the future to be skeptical of the results, but not of the decision itself.** This is the hardest part for me. We're all used to beating ourselves up for making "bad" decisions, but there's no such thing. No matter what you decide or how it turns out, there is information to be gained. So, choose a time in the future when you will assess your results without judgment. For almost every body-related goal (such as weight loss), four to six weeks is a good amount of time to gather data. During the decision-making process, choose the exact parameters you will consider a success, and then aim to meet that standard.

Here's how I see this play out for lots of women: You decide that your goal weight will be XXX pounds, because that number feels compelling and exciting right now. It's a little bit of a stretch, but not so much that you can't see yourself getting there. You've been that weight before—though not for quite a few years—and you're pretty sure that it will feel good in your body. You commit to finding your thoughts about that number and decide to think skeptically about your results in six weeks.

When the six-week mark rolls around, and you've lost just one pound and you're feeling defeated and frustrated, you think you need to change your goal weight. Maybe 175 is more realistic for you. Maybe your body has reached its set point. Maybe you're just never going to weigh what you want to weigh. Maybe your decision was a bad one.

NO!

Your goal weight decision is fine, but you're looking at the wrong results. It is such a common mistake to equate your "big picture" results with a "small picture" decision, as though they're related. This is something your brain does automatically and that you will want to become aware of, in order to use this decision-making process successfully.

Here's a much better example: You decide that your goal weight will be 150 pounds, because that number feels compelling and exciting right now. You create a goal statement for yourself of "I am losing weight until I reach 150 pounds," and have recognized that the feeling this thought creates for you is *motivation*. You commit to finding at least five thoughts every day for the next four weeks about your goal weight, with the task of deciding if they're helpful or unhelpful (using the Two-Step Tool). The result you are aiming for is to still feel motivation from your goal statement, or possibly some other helpful feeling, if not motivated.

At the end of four weeks, you pull out your journal to tally up how many thoughts you've found and to think skeptically about your results. You notice that even though you didn't journal every day, over the four weeks you still found more than twenty-three thoughts, and every single one of them was unhelpful. When you say your goal statement to yourself, you recognize that what you feel now is not motivation but *determination*. That is a good feeling, so you've met the standard you were aiming for.

Moving forward, you decide to ease up on the task of journaling every day—because, as it turns out, you don't make time for it on Mondays or Fridays—and commit to five days a week instead, while still finding at least twenty thoughts in the next four weeks. And at the end of four weeks, you take another skeptical look at these results to see if you're still feeling motivated, determined, or some other good feeling about your goal statement.

Now here's the thing: I know it feels unnatural to think so deliberately and to examine such a tiny sliver of what's going on in your life, as though you're putting a single cell under a microscope. It feels unnatural because it is! Your brain would much rather think of things in groups than as individual items. Certainly this makes sense given the plethora of information we're taking in at any given moment in time. If your brain didn't associate and categorize things quickly—and sometimes illogically—you wouldn't be able to process everything you're sensing.

What this means for you in a very practical, you're-gonna-want-to-look-for-this-while-journaling way is that you have unhelpful thoughts and remembered associations with specific numbers, like the last time you weighed your goal weight.

What I Weighed in Sixth Grade, on My Wedding Day, and at My Sister's Funeral

I know you know this, but I'll say it anyway: Your goal weight is a number, a factual and objective representation of the mass of your body in relation to gravity, as measured by a standardized device. Indeed, your goal weight as a number is an objective fact that could be provable in a court of law, if such a thing were needed. But your weight—both current and goal—is also a defining personal trait that gets displayed on your driver's license (in some states, like mine here in California), it's the subject of frequent conversations or just plain gossip about other people, and it's one of the ways we characterize ourselves in public or in the privacy of our own heads. The *fact* of our weight is that we *think* about our weight a lot. And yet, we hardly think about the *fact* of it at all because we are focusing on what our brain is making that number mean.

It's well studied and agreed upon that intense emotions help create lasting memories—this is why you remember exactly where you were and what you were doing on 9/11—and equally acknowledged as fact that our brains are constantly categorizing the information they receive from our senses, meaning what we see, touch, smell, taste, and feel in our bodies. When one of your sensory inputs for the day was seeing and acknowledging the number on the scale, it's no wonder that you can recall exactly what you weighed on the day you found out (and felt the intense emotions) about your husband cheating on you, or when you got that scary diagnosis, or—on a happier note—when your son got married.

One of my earliest associations with my weight is from childhood. My parents got divorced when I was in elementary school, and the summer before starting sixth grade, my mother, sister and I moved from Washington State to central California. That school year was tumultuous, as I navigated making new friends (and finding out who wasn't a friend) in unfamiliar surroundings with a drastically changed home life. I had been aware of my weight and my body before that, but sixth grade was when my brain started associating my weight with what I can now recognize as unrelated events.

I was up a couple of pounds the day my friend asked me to follow her into the bathroom, under the pretense of showing me "something gross," and then ran away when I complied, laughing and screaming about what a freak I was to a group of girls waiting outside. I was utterly mortified. The incident seemed to corroborate a fear deep inside of me that I was, at my core, unlikable and somehow just *made wrong*. The extreme emotion of that event has solidified the memory in my mind, and my brain—as it does—made the illogical connection between being heavier than normal and being socially ostracized.

The day I married my husband of (now) several decades was one of the happiest of my life, but many of the events leading up to and following the ceremony were filled with stress. We got married in a bit of a hurry—we had been engaged for a few months already and had begun planning a winter wedding, but our plans quickly changed during the first week of May when we decided to get married before the end of the month . . . on the *same day* we were both graduating from college, and that my husband was receiving his commission into the US Army. (Our rationale was, "Well, everybody's already going to be in town for the graduation and commissioning, we might as well get married, too." I still laugh every time I think of that!) And then the day after our wedding we moved to another state, hundreds of miles away from everybody and anything we'd ever known.

As it happened, I was the lightest I've ever been in my adult life on my wedding day, and even though I would rationally prefer to associate all the feel-good emotions of starting our new life together with being that weight, my brain followed its natural, biological behavioral patterns and homed straight in on all the negative emotions I felt in the weeks surrounding it. For years (until I uncovered the connection while I was journaling with the Two-Step Tool), my brain thought that being that particular weight equaled being stressed.

In 2016 and early 2017, I was the fittest, strongest, and fastest I have ever been. Over the course of about a year and a half, I ran a string of incredibly successful races that pushed me to my limits, including one of my longest races ever—100K—and my fastest finish times in the 5K, half marathon, and full marathon distances. I owed my success to finding my perfect racing weight and including regular strength training in my weekly routine. In May 2017, I was truly at the peak of my running and fitness game when my sister Vicki was diagnosed with terminal cancer. Just six and a half months later she was gone, I was devastated, and my brain started forming the illogical but biologically understandable hypothesis that when I am fit and strong and fast, people I love will die. Because brains think ridiculous things like that.

In hindsight, it's obvious that none of these events could possibly be related to my weight at the time when they happened, and that's exactly what I want to make clear: Your brain isn't logical! I mean, of course it is when you're thinking things on purpose, but our automatic thoughts (the ones in our subconscious that we don't hear until we go looking for them with our journal) are really running the show for our feelings and our actions, and thus, our results, and they're only capable of doing what biology dictates.

Your Goal Weight Feels Good

Let me be blunt: The actual number you choose doesn't matter even a tiny little bit. (That is, unless you choose a number that's unhealthily low.) Your goal weight is simply a measurement of your body's gravity. Of course you can calculate your BMI, or consult with your doctor, or Google some insurance charts that give you healthy weight ranges, but ultimately the decision is yours.

Here's my suggestion for how to choose: **Pick a number that feels good.** Because even though your goal weight is a number—factual data—you've just read ample evidence of how your brain is biologically destined to tell you a story about it, which means that your goal weight is a *thought.*

Yep. The sentence you hear in your head when you're thinking about what you want to weigh is a thought. And that means you can use the Two-Step Tool, which also means that you want a thought that feels good—helpful—in order to reach your goal. If the number you choose feels bad, it's not a helpful thought, and you're less likely to reach it as a goal.

When Are Your Thoughts a Problem?

As a weight-loss, fitness, and life coach, I've helped thousands of women find and manage their unhelpful thoughts on their way to a healthy weight. But sometimes unhelpful thoughts are disordered and you need more help than I can offer you. When this is the case, I wholeheartedly encourage you to seek it out. My rule of thumb for when it's time to look for personal, one-on-one professional help is . . . whenever you think you need it. Don't wait, and don't try to "handle things" on your own. Your mental health is important. Here are some of the signs I look for in my clients.

- Aiming for a weight goal that's lower than standard BMI or height-weight charts recommend

- Being overly concerned with one or two pounds of variation from the goal

> - Wanting to look a certain way much more than wanting to feel good or live an enjoyable life
> - Extreme restriction of food for nonmedical reasons
> - Rigidity of thinking (i.e., everything is black or white, right or wrong) or perfectionism
>
> These signs are subjective, and I don't believe that everybody with worries or concerns about their weight or food choices has disordered thinking. But if you're not sure, a consultation with a professional could be beneficial for you.

Let's Find Those RUTs

We're going to go through the Two-Step Tool a bit faster than in the last chapter, so if you need a refresher, be sure to head back to the last section of chapter 1 (page 23) for all the details. This was a particularly interesting journaling session for me, because I'm not trying to lose weight right now. So, just for fun, I chose the weight I was on my wedding day—which is a weight I haven't seen since 1996. Even though it's definitely not a current goal of mine, it's a weight I know my body is (technically) capable of being, so I didn't think I had any strong aversions to it. But boy, did my brain have some thoughts about that number!

And those thoughts did what all thoughts do—they created feelings. While I was writing, I felt the very strong urge to pick up my phone and check email in an attempt to avoid the churning of my stomach and the furrowing of my brow. I wanted to stop writing, to stop listening to these unpleasant thoughts, to just . . . *stop*. I mention this—and I'll continue to remind you of it every time we do this work—because I want to normalize it for you. Journaling and finding your unhelpful thoughts does not feel like getting licked by kittens. While you're doing it, it feels messy, it feels yucky, and it feels uncomfortable. There's rarely an immediate payoff, but there is a long-term benefit. In that sense, journaling is a lot like exercising—it doesn't always feel good in the moment, but you're always happy when you've gotten it done, and your health will improve over time. Here is my unfiltered journal entry, already updated with the phrase "I think" in front of each thought.

> **Journal Prompt: What do I think about weighing XXX?**

I think I can't get there.

I think that'll never happen.

I think I'll have to starve myself.

I think I'll look sick.

I think there's no way I can get that low.

I think I'm too different now.

I think there will be so many comments about my weight.

I think people already tell me I'm too thin.

I think I won't be able to hold on to that.

I think I'll gain it all back.

I think that's too low.

I think I'll have to give up dessert.

I think it'll be so hard.

I think I don't know how I can eat less than I do now.

I think I'm too heavy to get that skinny.

I think I was so young then.

I think people will tell me I look sickly.

As frequently happens when I'm writing my thoughts, I found myself agreeing with most of these statements as they came out of my pen. I mean, I *am* different now. I *was* young then. I *do* already get comments on social media about my weight. But even though my brain insists that these thoughts are true, that's not my objective here—I'm trying to find out if these thoughts are helpful for getting to my (alleged) goal weight, so next, I want to know how each thought makes me feel.

I think I can't get there. [Bad/Defeated]

I think that'll never happen. [Bad/Scornful]

I think I'll have to starve myself. [Bad/Deprived]

I think I'll look sick. [Bad/Embarrassed]

I think there's no way I can get that low. [Bad/Dismissive]

I think I'm too different now. [Bad/True/Sad]

I think there will be so many comments about my weight. [Bad/True/Reluctant]

I think people already tell me I'm too thin. [Bad/True/Annoyed]

I think I won't be able to hold on to that. [Bad/Defeated]

I think I'll gain it all back. [Bad/Resigned]

I think that's too low. [Bad/Unknown specific feeling]

I think I'll have to give up dessert. [Bad/Reluctant]

I think it'll be so hard. [Bad/True/Defeated]

I think I don't know how I can eat less than I do now. [Bad/Closed off]

I think I'm too heavy to get that skinny. [Bad/Unknown specific feeling]

I think I was so young then. [Bad/True/Wistful]

I think people will tell me I look sickly. [Bad/True/Annoyed]

I'm a pretty fast thinker, and often I am skipping a step or two ahead of myself when I'm doing something routine that I'm very familiar with. During my journaling with the Two-Step Tool, I deliberately and consciously slow myself down and take my time with each part of the process. Even though my brain would like to be all, "Yeah, yeah, yeah, these thoughts are unhelpful—let's go!" you can't "yeah, yeah, yeah" your way to making lasting changes in your life. So make sure you take the time to write UNHELPFUL next to every thought that created a bad feeling (whether you could identify the specific feeling or not—I don't always find a word that fits, and this work still has value).

I think I can't get there. [Bad/Defeated] UNHELPFUL

I think that'll never happen. [Bad/Scornful] UNHELPFUL

I think I'll have to starve myself. [Bad/Deprived] UNHELPFUL

I think I'll look sick. [Bad/Embarrassed] UNHELPFUL

I think there's no way I can get that low. [Bad/Dismissive] UNHELPFUL

I think I'm too different now. [Bad/True/Sad] UNHELPFUL

I think there will be so many comments about my weight. [Bad/True/Reluctant] UNHELPFUL

I think people already tell me I'm too thin. [Bad/True/Annoyed] UNHELPFUL

I think I won't be able to hold on to that. [Bad/Defeated] UNHELPFUL

I think I'll gain it all back. [Bad/Resigned] UNHELPFUL

I think that's too low. [Bad/Unknown specific feeling] UNHELPFUL

I think I'll have to give up dessert. [Bad/Reluctant] UNHELPFUL

I think it'll be so hard. [Bad/True/Defeated] UNHELPFUL

I think I don't know how I can eat less than I do now. [Bad/Closed off] UNHELPFUL

I think I'm too heavy to get that skinny. [Bad/Unknown Specific feeling] UNHELPFUL

I think I was so young then. [Bad/True/Wistful] UNHELPFUL

I think people will tell me I look sickly. [Bad/True/Annoyed] UNHELPFUL

Your Turn: Quick Practice and More Journal Prompts

You've been doing a great job absorbing all this information and practicing with the quick journal prompts. How do I know? Because you're still here. If you're reading these words, you're on the right track and making terrific progress. So let's do a little "readiness assessment" to see what you're thinking about your goals. Get a piece of paper and something to write with, and let's find **one thought: What do I think about setting a weight-loss goal?**

You know the drill—write down whatever just popped in your head, even if it doesn't seem related. That sentence is a thought, so write "I think" in front of it. Read it to yourself out loud: "I *think* . . ." How do you feel when you think that thought? Write HELPFUL next to your thought if it feels good, or UNHELPFUL next to it if it feels bad.

I'm hard-pressed to think of a topic in your life where you will achieve all of the self-awareness available to you with a "one and done" journaling session—meaning that you are likely to want to come at any topic you choose from a variety of angles to find more (let's be honest, probably unhelpful) thoughts. When you're ready for them, here are some suggestions for finding more thoughts about your goal weight.

- What do I think about the last time I weighed XXX?

- What do I think weighing XXX will feel like?

- What do I think I'll have to do when I weigh XXX?

- What do I think other people will think of me when I weigh XXX?

- What do I think about other women who weigh XXX?

- What do I think is the problem with weighing XXX?

Borrow This (Possibly) Helpful Thought

Remember that you absolutely don't need to force a helpful thought into your head, nor is this automatically going to be a helpful thought for you. Rather, give this some consideration and ask yourself how you feel when you say it: **I am a person who weighs XXX [your goal weight].**

I'm going to guess that on your first pass, what you feel is disbelief, right? Because of course you're not currently a person who weighs your goal weight, that's why it's a goal weight! But hear me out here: The phrase "I am" is the most powerful in human language, bringing an immediacy to whatever follows it—and it doesn't have to be taken literally. We use that phrase to describe our jobs, our hobbies, as well as our mood or other transitory feelings like hunger or tiredness, and yet we know that it is not a description of our complete selves. "I am happy" doesn't imply that you are only happy, or that you are always happy every minute of every day, or that happy is the only thing you can be. It means you *feel* happy, right now. What if you *feel* like a person who weighs your goal weight? What would that feel like? Good? If this moment of imagining yourself at your goal weight feels good, then this is a helpful thought. (And if not, then it's unhelpful and you can disregard it.) In fact, if imagining yourself at your goal weight feels good, this is an incredibly helpful thought, because it's priming your brain for success. Daydreaming (or *prospection*, if you'd like a fancier word for it) isn't just an idle use of your time.

The part of your brain that will get you out of bed for your early morning workout, or plan and prep meals on the weekends, or reach your hand for the water bottle again and again is motivated by imagination, because it's not making the distinction between reality and fantasy. When you picture yourself in the future, weighing your goal weight and doing the things you want to do, you are creating feelings of confidence and certainty right now that will, in turn, drive your actions today.

To your brain, while you are imagining yourself at your goal weight, you *are* your goal weight, so of course you will do all the things—such as managing your mind, eating right, exercising regularly, drinking water, and sleeping adequately—that a person at that weight would do.

Scale Thoughts: Weighing Yourself Daily

Remember that a thought is our brain's interpretation of facts, so when you step on the scale and see a number, your brain is *automatically* turning that number into a story. That's what brains do. And the story your brain is telling you about that number (or the number of your goal weight, or the number of pounds you'd like to lose, or the number of pounds you've already lost, or the number of pounds that girl you don't even know in real life but you follow her on Instagram has lost in less time than you) is based on your perception of past experiences, as well as thoughts and ideas you've been exposed to in the media and through interactions with other people. Your brain is then running that story through all of its biological filters, too—wanting to stay alive and stay the same, believing the worst of a situation, and finding evidence to agree with itself.

No wonder it feels so dramatic when you step on the scale! You're not just looking at a number and seeing it as data, you're replaying years of old, potentially unhelpful messages in your head. Today's weight is burdened with every thought you've ever had about your weight. This is why you don't want to weigh yourself every day (or every week, or *ever*). It feels like an onslaught of thoughts and feelings and just—UGH! But here I am, suggesting that the path to weight-loss success is paved with **daily weigh-ins.**

Do I really have to weigh myself every day?

No, you don't. In fact, when it comes to following my—or anybody's—weight-loss advice: You never *have to* do anything. There are two good reasons why. First, let's quickly run that sentence through the Two-Step Tool and see if it's a helpful thought. How do you feel when you say, "I have to . . ." anything, not just weighing yourself? For me, the phrase *have to* almost always feels bad, like pressure or obligation or abject resignation. So "I have to . . ." is not likely going to be a thought that gets you where you want to go. And second, you have agency over any program you choose to participate in, including the 5-0 Method and the advice in this book. Take in the information, decide what works for you—by using the Two-Step Tool, if you like it!—and disregard the rest.

Coming back to the question at hand, *yes*, it's my suggestion that you weigh yourself every day, because the scale is an area of weight loss that is rife with opportunities to find your thoughts. That said, there are options for how often to weigh yourself, based on your current thoughts and feelings about weighing yourself (more on this in a little bit). Let's look at three distinct parts of weighing yourself where you can use the Two-Step Tool.

1. **The idea of being weighed, in general.** For many women, the notion of getting on a scale *at all*—let alone every day—feels overwhelming. Depending on the specific thoughts you have, you might feel angry, defensive, skeptical, or just generally *bad* about the possibility of being confronted with the data of your weight.

2. **The anticipation of weighing in.** I have worked with many women who experience "scale anxiety" in the days or hours before weighing themselves. You might feel like you're tying yourself in knots, worrying about what number will show up.

3. **After seeing your weight.** Even if you feel fine about the idea of weighing in, and don't seem to mind the act of stepping on the scale, once there's a number showing between your feet—well, then your brain has some things to say to you.

The Pros and Cons of Exposure Therapy (Systematic Desensitization)

Because of social conditioning, there's a pretty good chance that, right now on some level, you're equating your weight with your moral character or your worthiness. Most people have some version of an "ideal body type," and anybody who is outside that norm is likely to have unhelpful thoughts about themselves. For many Western women in particular, these unhelpful thoughts manifest as fears, worries, and anxieties about their weight and the scale. (Briefly let me state for the record that **your weight means absolutely nothing about who you are as a human being.** You are, regardless of your physical vessel, a completely whole, completely lovable, and completely worthy person whose value is not predicated on your body.)

The point of weighing yourself every day—and the reason I recommend it—is to learn how to see the numbers as data. In fact, ultimately, I'd like for you to learn how to see your weight as good, useful data that corroborates your progress, and eventually confirms the successful achievement of reaching your goal weight.

Okay, Pahla . . . but how?

Through a specific therapeutic learning protocol called exposure therapy. In the early and mid-1900s, when psychology was still clearly delineated into the separate camps of behaviorism and cognition, behavioral researchers experimented with so-called *counterconditioning*, in an effort to cure patients of their anxieties and phobias. The idea was that repeated exposure to a specific fear in a controlled environment where the patient was rewarded for engaging with the object of fear would reduce or eliminate that phobia. In modern times, there are numerous types of protocols for desensitization therapy that include not just the act of exposure but also the simultaneous use of somatic and cognitive tools such as relaxation breathing and listing anxiety-producing thoughts (journaling).

The truth of it is that simply exposing yourself frequently to something that you have unhelpful thoughts about isn't enough to change those unhelpful thoughts. As we've seen throughout this book, neuroplasticity—changing your thoughts—requires you to be aware of the thoughts you want to change and actively requesting your brain to recategorize them (exactly what we do with the Two-Step Tool—find your thoughts and decide if they're helpful).

Time to Find Those RUTs

What if you have so many Really Unhelpful Thoughts about weighing yourself that you just . . . *can't even* (as the kids say)? As in, what if you have unhelpful thoughts about the scale in general, coupled with daily scale anxiety, and then you pile on the flood of thoughts about the number you're seeing every morning?

In conditions like that, you're likely to simply quit weighing yourself altogether (and possibly even give up your quest to find a healthy weight). Rather than jumping into the deep end of the "weighing yourself daily" pool and hoping you can learn to swim before you sink, let's use the Two-Step Tool to help you decide where to start.

> **Journal Prompt: What do I think about weighing myself, ever?**

Our first question is much broader than I usually suggest, and that's on purpose. We're simply gauging how you feel about scales and weighing yourself in the most general sense. Imagine yourself approaching a scale with the intention of getting on it. What do you think?

This one was relatively easy for me because I have been doing my own work on the scale for quite some time (and you can get to this point, too, if you're not already). I found four helpful thoughts, and then my brain started to get bored with the question. Here's my completed journal entry, with all parts of the Two-Step Tool finished.

I think it's fine. [Good/Accepting] HELPFUL

I think it's interesting information. [Good/Curious] HELPFUL

I think I like keeping track. [Good/Organized] HELPFUL

I think I like how much I weigh. [Good/Loving] HELPFUL

(Now, I moved through the Two-Step Tool process like lightning in this section, but if you need a refresher on how to use the Two-Step Tool, jump back to chapter 1, page 23.)

STOP HERE and do not move on to any sort of weighing activity if you didn't find any helpful thoughts. Your exposure therapy starts with simply imagining yourself near a scale with the intention of weighing yourself and using the Two-Step Tool on your thoughts. Repeat this process daily—or at least frequently—until you find a minimum of one helpful thought.

Remember that your imagination helps to prime your brain for success because your brain doesn't distinguish between reality and fantasy. The same principle applies here with imaginary exposure to the fearful object—you're gently exposing yourself to the scale in a safe and controlled way that can help open up your brain to other thought options over time.

MOVE ON to the next question when you find one or more help-ful thoughts, because that's where we're going to decide how often you're ready to weigh yourself.

> **Journal Prompt: What do I think about weighing myself every day?**

You're going to use your imagination again and ask this question of yourself in a theoretical way. What do you think *it would be like* to weigh yourself every day? (Because you're going to have the oppor-tunity to explore what it *is* like once you start doing it.) If you find helpful thoughts right away, this might be a short journaling session for you, but don't worry if it takes some time. Being patient and al-lowing your brain to tell you what it's thinking is an essential skill to develop for deep self-awareness.

My helpful to unhelpful thought ratio for this question was still quite high—again, because I've done this work over the last few years, but before that it was all unhelpful—so I'll move through the Two-Step Tool quickly. Nearly all of my thoughts about daily weigh-ins are helpful. Here's my completed journal entry, with all parts of the Two-Step Tool finished.

I think I like the information. [Good/Open or Accepting] HELPFUL

I think it's part of my routine. [Good/True/Satisfied] HELPFUL

I think I like to know more than not knowing. [Good/Curious]
HELPFUL

I think it's fine. [Good/Unknown specific feeling] HELPFUL

I think other people might think it's too much. [Bad/Defensive]
HELPFUL

I think it's good information. [Good/Accepting] HELPFUL

STOP HERE and revise the journal prompt if you didn't have any helpful thoughts. Adjust the question to "What do I think about weighing myself every other day (or once a week, or every other week, or once a month, or whatever amount of time seems like it might work for you)?" and use the Two-Step Tool until you find a minimum of one helpful thought.

MOVE ON to the next step when you've found one or more helpful thoughts. Your exposure therapy starts by using the interval of weighing yourself where you found the one (or several) helpful thought(s).

> ### Journal Prompt: What do I think
> ### about today's weight?

And now the fun really begins when you start to collect the data of your regular weigh-ins! This question is multipurpose and could be used both before and after stepping on the scale if you are interested in finding all of those thoughts. That might sound like a lot of journaling, but it doesn't have to take more than a minute or two. You don't need to agonize over finding every single thought. Truly, you can gain a surprising amount of insight by finding just one or two thoughts at a time.

This morning, before hopping on the scale, I took a moment to jot down a couple of thoughts I heard rattling around in my brain.

It's going to be higher.

I probably ate too much yesterday.

I don't think I slept enough.

Let's take the time to go through the Two-Step Tool fully on this one and notice the "worry thoughts" your brain might have in anticipation of stepping on the scale. Worrying is your brain trying to predict the future (which it can't possibly know), so these are going to be unhelpful thoughts, but let's pop a little "I think" in front of each of those sentences to recognize them as automatic, efficient impulses of electricity running through your brain that are subject to the demands of biology (including negativity bias and confirmation bias).

I think it's going to be higher.

I think I probably ate too much yesterday.

I think I don't think I slept enough.

Next up, let's determine what kind of feeling is created when you think each thought.

I think it's going to be higher. [Bad/Worried]

I think I probably ate too much yesterday. [Bad/Judged/Ashamed]

I think I don't think I slept enough. [Bad/Frustrated]

And finally, it's time to write UNHELPFUL next to each sentence to help your brain recategorize these thoughts, so it can get less efficient at thinking them.

> *I think* it's going to be higher. [Bad/Worried] UNHELPFUL
>
> *I think* I probably ate too much yesterday. [Bad/Judged/Ashamed] UNHELPFUL
>
> *I think* I don't think I slept enough. [Bad/Frustrated] UNHELPFUL

Now, you might be thinking to yourself right about now, "Pahla, I don't get it. You've done all this work on your thoughts about weighing yourself, so why do you still worry before you get on the scale?" This is a great question, and I'll answer it with an example from my time as a preschool teacher.

The beautiful art of gentle redirection

Let me start by giving you a little bit of what you might initially think of as "bad news": Your brain is always going to offer you unhelpful thoughts. But—here comes the good news—after you've been finding your thoughts for a while and deciding if they're helpful, you'll start to recognize the familiar troublemakers that are always turning up. Or, as I think of them after five years of being a preschool teacher—*naughty children.* (Let me clarify that every child who was ever in my care was a darling, cherubic angel that I adored like my very own . . . but some of them required more attention than others.)

As I mentioned in chapter 2, likening your automatic thoughts to small children is completely apropos: They're illogical, stubborn, and have zero attention span or social skills. They can be loud and demanding or silent and sullen. They get crankier when they're tired or hungry, and you never know when they're going to surprise you with a sudden burst of loving tenderness. And also—the best thing about both small kiddos and your automatic, efficient thoughts—they're easily distracted.

When little Sparky starts to get grabby hands and doesn't want to share with the other kids, all you have to do is gently redirect him to a different toy (preferably across the room) that he can play with on his own for a minute or two. And when he gets tired of that, he'll move on to something else.

Remember how asking a question always grabs your attention? This trick works especially well with your unhelpful worries and little ones, too. I like to make the question sound especially exciting and fun, as though the new thing we're going to play with/think about is soooooo much better than the one we've already got.

"Sparky, I see that you're throwing the crayons at Sally's face, but did you know that there's magical squishy dough at the other play table?" is akin to "Brain, I totally agree that my weight could go up today, but did you know that there's also a chance it could go down or stay the same?"

Yes, I still have "worry thoughts," even though I have directed my brain to label them as UNHELPFUL, but after years of recognizing them for what they are and feeling all the way through the feelings they create—a super fun skill we're going to explore in the very next chapter—I don't actually *feel* the worry. I can simply hear the thought and gently redirect it. And, yes, I absolutely use my "preschool teacher voice" when doing so.

Normal Daily Weight Fluctuations Are Part of the Game

Yesterday's weight was down by over half a pound, but today's is up nearly a pound and a half—what's going on with that? Is it because you ate something salty last night, or are you gaining weight? Have you been eating too many calories or not exercising enough? Or—even though this still sounds impossible—could it be that you're exercising too much and eating too little? It could be one of those things or none of them!

The fact is, your body weight is constantly fluctuating because of the billions of processes going on in your body all day long, every day, for your entire life. The weight you see on the scale reflects not just what you had to eat or drink yesterday, but also how much sleep you've gotten recently, how much stress or inflammation you have, and possibly whether you have food waste that hasn't been evacuated yet (yes, the scale might be up because you need to poop).

Use the Two-Step Tool on your thoughts about fluctuations—there's a good chance that most of what you're thinking isn't helpful. When you can see a downward trend over time, you *are* losing weight successfully!

> **Journal Prompt: What do I think about today's weight (after the weigh-in)?**

Are you ready to feel angry, frustrated, disappointed, infuriated, crushed, or defeated? Because those are some of the exciting emotions that might be waiting for you to discover in your journal after you weigh yourself. So let's dig in! Recently, I've been having fabulous thoughts about my weight, so I went searching through some "archival footage"—my old journals—to share some of the unhelpful thoughts I've noticed on my way to finding helpful ones.

Here's my raw journal entry from several years ago, already updated with "I think" and the feeling each thought created for me:

I think I hate it! [Bad/Furious]

I think I'm out of control. [Bad/Helpless]

I think I can't stand this. [Bad/Burdened]

I think I've never been this fat before. [Bad/Dramatic]

I think I'm eating too much. [Bad/Shameful]

I think I have to get ahold of myself. [Bad/Out of control]

I think I have to stop snacking. [Bad/Pressured]

I think I need to get control. [Bad/Helpless]

I think it's so much. [Bad/Burdened]

I think I can't believe I let myself get here again. [Bad/Scorn]

I think I must be eating too much. [Bad/Judged]

Even reading these words from a stranger, you're probably feeling some of the gut-churning anger and impotent helplessness of these thoughts. Let me tell you, not a single one of these thoughts were helpful in getting me to my goal weight. But my brain didn't know that until I told it so.

Take the time to compassionately notice how painful your thoughts are, and how much they're holding you back. You have the power to change your mind. You have to ability to direct your brain to think new things. And it starts by labeling your current thoughts as UNHELPFUL.

I think I hate it! [Bad/Furious] UNHELPFUL

I think I'm out of control. [Bad/Helpless] UNHELPFUL

I think I can't stand this. [Bad/Burdened] UNHELPFUL

I think I've never been this fat before. [Bad/Dramatic] UNHELPFUL

I think I'm eating too much. [Bad/Shameful] UNHELPFUL

I think I have to get ahold of myself. [Bad/Out of control] UNHELPFUL

I think I have to stop snacking. [Bad/Pressured] UNHELPFUL

I think I need to get control. [Bad/Helpless] UNHELPFUL

I think it's so much. [Bad/Burdened] UNHELPFUL

I think I can't believe I let myself get here again. [Bad/Scorn] UNHELPFUL

I think I must be eating too much. [Bad/Judged] UNHELPFUL

Borrow This (Possibly) Helpful Thought

Can you picture a time when you'll think your weight is amazing? Maybe after you get to your goal weight? But what if you thought that *right now*? You can borrow this (possibly) helpful thought and start thinking it immediately, no matter what number shows up on the scale each day: **This is exactly what I wanted.**

I can see how you might think this thought is preposterous. "But Pahla," you're shouting at me through the pages, "this *isn't even close* to what I wanted to weigh today!" But what if it is? What if you felt so completely certain that your goal weight is coming to you in the future that today's weight seems like the exact place you're supposed to be on this journey? And what if what you really want, as much as your goal weight, is to feel loving and accepting of yourself?

What does it feel like when you say, "This is exactly what I wanted" to yourself? If you're struggling with it, try picturing yourself receiving a just-right gift—the thing you didn't even know you needed but you're now excited to have. For me, in a word, this thought creates the feeling of *contentedness*.

If that's not where you are right now, and this thought feels lousy, then out the window it goes, because it's unhelpful for you.

Everything We Learned in This Chapter

- Having a specific goal in mind is crucial to success.

- Making a decision requires three steps: Make the decision, commit to finding your thoughts about the decision, and be skeptical about the results at a specific time in the future but not of the decision itself.

- You have automatic, illogical associations with your goal weight that are unhelpful.

- You can choose your goal weight simply because the number feels good.

- There are a variety of possible questions to ask yourself when you're finding your thoughts on any topic.

- Your brain is not thinking in facts, it is interpreting facts and telling you a story.

- Weighing yourself is the fastest (but not necessarily the easiest or best) way to find your thoughts about the scale.

- Exposure therapy is a useful tool for reducing the fear or anxiety of weighing yourself.

- Recurring "worry thoughts" can be acknowledged as unhelpful and gently redirected.

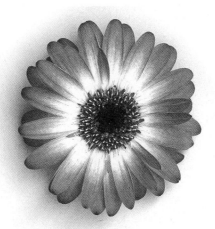

PART THREE

Loving Your Body

CHAPTER 5

Menopause Changed So Much More Than Your Periods

Loving Your Body

Here's the truth: Losing weight won't make you happy with your body. Or happy in general. We know that our thoughts create our feelings, and we've explored how the thoughts you are currently having are creating lots of unpleasant feelings, and that's how you know that those thoughts are unhelpful in your quest to lose weight. Even so, there might still be a part of you that thinks you'll be happy *because* you've lost all the weight—and that part of you is wrong.

Your feelings are always created by your thoughts rather than the circumstances of your weight, shape, fitness, or health. You've almost certainly seen examples of how people with amazing-seeming circumstances aren't happy. Think of celebrities who are miserable even though they're beautiful and famous and have lots of money, or women you know who have fantastic bodies and still complain about how they feel unattractive.

Let me be clear that even though losing weight won't *make you* happy, being a healthy weight has numerous benefits, not the least of which are having energy, and living a long, healthy life. The journey of working toward and then achieving your healthy weight is also immensely beneficial because it will teach you so much about yourself, your body, and your ability to do anything you set your mind to. But having the body of your dreams won't automatically generate love for your body.

The way to love your body is to think *thoughts* that create *feelings* of love. On the one hand, this task sounds quite simple. And, technically, it is—you're capable of thinking loving thoughts about your body right now in the same way that you're capable of thinking anything. But on the other hand, as we've seen in the previous chapters, there's a good chance you have some not-so-helpful automatic thoughts about menopause and how different your body is, during and after the change.

It's no wonder you have unhelpful thoughts about menopause and your menopausal body when you're surrounded by negative images, stories, and language about this transition. TV shows and movies have normalized the idea that menopause is a miserable time in a woman's life; advertisers want to sell you lotions, creams, and supplements to "reverse aging;" and even some medical professionals use phrases like "estrogen deficiency" or "ovarian failure" to describe menopause. Your body is neither deficient nor failing, you don't have to feel miserable, and the process of aging is not only natural but full of opportunities to understand yourself on a deeper level.

There's No Turning Back

One of the most common sentiments I hear from women I work with—and the thing I said myself when menopause came knocking at my door and changed my body in ways I didn't understand at the time—is that they want to "get back to" feeling like themselves, or a weight they used to be. Even though you understand that time moves only in one direction—forward—your brain still offers you the known quantity of your past weight or past fitness as a target that you can aim for. While this might seem harmless on its surface, let me point out that "getting back to your old body" when menopause has fundamentally changed nearly every process in your body is a goal that's *impossible* to achieve, and thus a waste of your time.

To illustrate this, let's quickly run that sentence "I want to get back to feeling like I used to" through the Two-Step Tool. First, recognize that this is just a thought—"I *think* I want to get back to feeling like I used to." That pulled the "truthiness" away from it a little, didn't it? Now, how do you feel when you think "I want to get back to feeling like I used to?" My immediate response to this question was *desperate*. Desperate feels like a sinking feeling in my stomach and an emptiness in my chest—so this is not a good feeling. So, "I want to get back to feeling like I used to" is unhelpful for reaching my goal of loving my menopausal body.

Rather than aiming to re-create your past self, your best bet is to get informed about what's going on with your body right now, so you can intentionally create your best self and live happily into the future.

Estrogen Has Changed Your Heart, Muscles, Bones, Brain, and Balance

We've explored (in chapters 2 and 3) how declining estrogen has affected weight loss and made conditions easier for weight gain, but now it's time to dive into the health-related changes your body is experiencing. Even though you might have been taught from a young age to focus on your appearance, your health is significantly more important. Finding a healthy weight will be of great benefit to your overall health, with far fewer of the risks associated with obesity. Even more than being healthy, changes to your exercise routine (which are fueled by changes in your thinking) can help you toward your ultimate goal of truly loving your body.

Estrogen and your heart

Among the many things estrogen has been doing all these years that was easy to take for granted is protecting you from heart disease by keeping your blood vessels supple and flexible. In combination with the other changes your body could be undergoing from dwindling estrogen and chronically elevated cortisol—such as increased abdominal fat, insulin resistance, general weight gain, elevated blood sugar, and higher blood pressure—this change to your blood vessels can put you at significant risk for sudden stroke, chronic heart disease, and even heart failure.

There's a good chance you've worried about the men in your life having a heart attack, but the truth is that cardiovascular disease is the number one cause of death for women, and nearly as many women as men die of heart-related illnesses every year. (According to the CDC, over three hundred thousand women in the US alone die every year of heart disease, with another one hundred thousand dying of stroke and other hypertensive issues.)

If you already enjoy cardio exercises such as walking, swimming, golfing, gardening, cycling, using an elliptical machine, or running, then keeping your heart healthy will be a breeze. However, if the idea of sweating and breathing heavy is a "hard pass" for you, this will require some adjustments to your routine and your mindset (which we'll get into on page 148).

Estrogen and your muscles

During the menopause transition, you lose muscle mass, strength, and tone faster than at any other point in your life. Not only was estrogen helping you recover from your workouts properly, but your ovaries also used to produce more testosterone, which has been important all these years for muscle growth and maintenance. The decline in these hormones, along with an increase in cortisol, has a profound and compounding effect on your body composition—the decreased muscle mass reduces your metabolic rate, making it easier to gain fat. Put simply, muscles burn more calories than other tissue, so fewer muscles means a lower overall burn rate.

You may first notice these changes by the way your body looks, but it isn't just an aesthetic issue. Having less muscle mass means you aren't as physically strong as you once were, and it means your bones are less protected from falls.

For many women, the idea of picking up weights feels either intimidating or uninteresting. I used to belong in that camp myself—until I started lifting weights at home and realized that it's just as fun as cardio. If you already enjoy using dumbbells, there's a good chance your menopausal muscle tone isn't in danger. But if you're not yet a fan, you'll want to examine your thoughts and your routine.

Estrogen and your bones

You were told to drink milk to build strong bones, but in truth, protecting and maintaining your bone health was also one of estrogen's jobs. While there's more research to be done, scientists have concluded that estrogen is responsible for regulating the entire bone life cycle—meaning, the creation of new bone, maintenance of existing bone, and resorption of old bone cells back into the body. There's some evidence that a lack of estrogen correlates with elevated levels of bone resorption and reduced production of osteoblasts (the cells that form new bone). This is to say that during the menopause transition and afterward, you are losing bone density faster than you are creating it.

The weakening of your bones puts you at risk of fractures—particularly of the hip, wrist, and spine—and the complications (not to mention costs) that accompany them. While osteoporosis is not a deadly disease, it is insidious and painful, robbing its sufferers of quality of life rather than quantity. Thankfully, the fix for bone density issues is the same as for building muscle tone, which we'll get to on page 150.

Estrogen and your brain

Brain fog and memory lapses are common symptoms of menopause that may be linked to diminishing estrogen. Some studies indicate that estrogen has had a protective effect on brain function and cognition that can lead to memory loss during menopause. While the reasons for it are unclear, women are far more likely to develop Alzheimer's disease or dementia than men. Loss of memory and cognitive function are not—in and of themselves—fatal, but these conditions severely restrict your quality of life.

There's ample evidence that an overall healthy lifestyle, including adequate nutrition and hydration, restorative sleep, reduction of stress, and consistent exercise can reduce your risk of developing neurocognitive disorders. The type of exercise doesn't make a difference, so when you create a balanced routine for your bones, muscles, heart, and lungs—you'll be doing good things for your brain, too.

Estrogen and your balance

While a reduction in estrogen doesn't affect your balance directly, it is correlated with an increased stiffness in tendons and ligaments, which—combined with reduced muscle mass, brain fog, or other somatic symptoms such as hot flashes—could have the effect of worsening your balance as you age. And a lack of balance greatly increases your risk of falling. While falling might not seem serious—most people who fall will survive—it comes with a risk of complications, such as sepsis, brain injury, or loss of independence. For women over sixty-five, falling is the leading cause of accidental death.

It's simple to include balance exercises in your daily route—such as standing on one foot for a short period of time. If you already enjoy balancing, you're doing great. But if the thought of practicing your balance has you sweating more than cardio, then you'll want to make the adjustments to your routine and your mindset that I recommend on page 148.

You Don't Need to Balance Your Hormones, but You Do Need to Balance Your Exercise Program

There's an entire industry of supplement suppliers and saliva-test-kit makers who would love for you to worry about balancing your hormones, but your body will do this all on its own if you concentrate on balancing your lifestyle activities. Without your pre-menopausal levels of estrogen around to protect your heart, build your muscles, keep your bones strong, and help you stay on your feet, it's now up to *you* to create a lifestyle routine that promotes heart health, strength, brain function, and balance. In return for your consistent, moderate efforts, your body and hormones will balance themselves.

One of the five things we do each day to lose weight with the 5-0 Method is to exercise moderately (which we discussed in chapter 3). I suspect that, left to your own devices, you'll choose your favorite activity most days of the week and then throw in some of the workouts you don't really care for once in a while, right? Me, too. Sign me up for cardio every day! While it's true that you can lose weight this way, if you want *all* the benefits of working out—visible muscle tone, increased stamina and energy, and the functional fitness to enjoy yourself well into old age—you're going to want to be a little more strategic than that.

My suggestion: **A healthy and well-rounded weekly exercise routine includes four days of cardiovascular activity, three days of strength-building activity, and balance practice every day.**

Much as you might like cardio to do everything for you, it alone isn't going to get you those Michelle Obama arms or help you get back up off the floor after you pull the wrapping paper storage bin out from under your bed.

A Quick Word About Meeting the CDC's Exercise Guidelines

The CDC recommends that adults of all ages aim for 150 minutes per week of moderate-intensity aerobic activity, plus two sessions per week of muscle-building activity. Here we'll clarify how the 5-0 Method meets the CDC guidelines while getting you to your healthy weight *and* reaping optimum health benefits.

How can you squeeze everything the CDC wants you to do into a daily 23-minute weight-loss workout? In a word: MetCon.

Okay, technically, MetCon is short for two words—Metabolic Conditioning—which is a workout that alternates between cardio and strength, with little or no rest between exercises, to keep your heart beating at a moderately aerobic rate. And if you'd like two more words for a workout that does double duty in your optimal heart rate range, there's also Cardio Toning, which is a fast-paced, cardio-style workout using your lightest weights.

So, why do I recommend three days of strength work in the 5-0 Method? Shouldn't one of them be another cardio day? Nope. Because of a fun little thing called "cardiac drift."

In a nutshell, cardiac drift means that over time, even with very little exercise exertion, your heart rate will naturally rise. So, even a slow-moving strength workout—which, by the way, is significantly more than "very little exercise exertion" when you're using moderately heavy dumbbells—will increase your heart rate to the recommended range.

Once we add in the 5-0 Method's built-in daily balance work (which the CDC doesn't even mention until you are over sixty-five years old), you are actually *exceeding* the CDC's guidelines and getting a beautifully balanced 161 minutes of exercise each week.

Why (and how) cardio is good for your heart and lungs

Our brain and body adhere to several biological imperatives (rules): Number one is to stay alive, number two is to reproduce, and numbers three and four—the ones we'll focus on here—are to stay the same as much as possible (to expend as little energy as it needs to) and to make adaptations when necessary. This fourth imperative exists because of the third one. When you exercise, you are expending more energy than when you're resting, and while your body is fine with doing so, it's still keeping a frugal eye on your energy stores. It has systems in place to make sure that the work you're doing won't be as "expensive" the next time you do it.

Let's say you go for a brisk walk. While you're walking, your heart and lungs are both working harder and faster than at rest, because your muscles need more oxygenated blood than while you're doing nothing. This is hard work for your heart and lungs, so after your walk, your body initiates a complex chemical and hormonal re-sponse that strengthens the heart muscle, improves vascular flow rates, increases lung capacity, and strengthens your breathing mus-cles. Over time, with regular workouts, you will be able to take in more oxygen, your heart will pump harder, and your veins will deliv-er more blood to the farthest reaches of your body—as well as return that blood quicker—all with the same effort as before. In short, your body adapts so that its energy output can stay the same.

Why (and how) strength training is good for your muscles and bones

This basic principle of making adaptations in order to stay the same applies to all types of exercise and body systems, including your musculoskeletal system. Interestingly, improvements to your mus-cle mass and bone density are intrinsically linked because the mech-anism by which you increase muscle mass—with resistance work, like strength training with dumbbells—also builds bone density.

Your muscles are attached to your bones (with tendons and ligaments) because they need to work together to produce body movement. Without bones, your muscles would have no form or structure; and without muscles, your bones wouldn't be able to move. When you exercise, you are placing stress on both your mus-cles and bones at the same time. And in response to this stress, your body initiates the chemical and hormonal processes that repair your muscles and bones by making them thicker and denser—and capable of doing more work with the same amount of energy output.

Why (and how) balance training is good for your brain and your body

Improving your balance is proof that your brain—along with your muscles and bones—will make adaptations when prompted. Regular exercise has been shown to improve cognitive function, reduce the risk of neurocognitive disease, and promote neuroplasticity. Good balance depends on your body and brain working in tandem with your *proprioception*, which is an internal awareness of where your body is and how it is moving. And the only way to strengthen this awareness is to practice. A little balance practice goes a long way. In just a few weeks you can see (and feel) dramatic changes in your movement patterns and ability to balance with less than five minutes of practice each day.

But good for you doesn't mean you want to do it

Have you ever noticed how big the gap can be between "good for you" and "what you do in your daily life"? Because it's huge! If we were all doing what was good for us, life would certainly be simpler. But we've all had habits normalized for us—smoking, drinking, overeating, and plenty of others—that feel comfortable, familiar, and pleasurable even if they're not in our best health interests. But remember, the only reason your current habits *feel* comfortable, familiar, and pleasurable is because you have *thoughts* about them. Which means that you're very likely to have not-so-comfortable, not-so-familiar, and not-so-pleasurable thoughts about changing your routine to accommodate the changes of menopause. And those are the thoughts that are slowing you down.

Remember that your brain is always seeking pleasure and avoiding pain. So, it stands to reason that when you have pleasurable thoughts about eating or exercising or sleeping the way you've always done (and painful, or at least unpleasant, thoughts about making changes), you'll continue on the familiar path. This is the exact reason why you're learning to examine your thoughts with the Two-Step Tool—so you can create healthy changes in your life, instead of continuing to do the same old thing, by becoming aware of the thoughts that are driving your current actions. So, let's get out our journals and start exploring!

When I went looking through my old journal entries, I didn't have to go back very far. This work on loving my body through the menopausal change has been ongoing for several years, and brought with it some of the most difficult—and also satisfying!—mindset shifts in my life.

> **Journal Prompt: What do I think about changing my routine for menopause?**

I don't want to.

I hate that my body is different now.

I wish I could stay the same.

I don't want to change.

I don't know what to do.

I hate this different body.

Menopause sucks.

I don't want to.

I have to be so careful about everything now.

I don't want to think so hard.

I like my routine the way it is.

I want to keep doing what I've been doing.

THIS SHOULDN'T BE HAPPENING TO ME!

We now interrupt our regularly scheduled Two-Step Tool . . .

As soon as that last sentence left my pen, I put it down and started sobbing. This thought (which we'll work on identifying and really recognizing it as a thought in a bit) felt so real and so painful that it required immediate attention, in the form of feeling this feeling all the way through.

What's a Feeling, Anyway?

Feelings are a cascade of hormonal reactions—triggered by the neuroelectric impulse of a thought—that result in such changes to your body as clammy skin, an elevated heart rate, increased blood flow that creates a tingling sensation, a quickness to your breathing, or dryness in your mouth. Without intervention, the physical effects of feelings last about 90 seconds before they dissipate. They are completely natural and, in fact, you are *designed* to feel them. Biologically speaking, your feelings exist to give you information and propel you into action. Remember that every result in your life stems from this chain of events: Your thoughts create your feelings, then your feelings drive your actions.

Throughout history feelings have been viewed as less useful than rational thought, but nothing could be further from the truth. Without feelings, you wouldn't *do* anything, so you wouldn't create any results in your life. And I'm not just talking about big results like making a million dollars or losing a hundred pounds, I mean even something as simple as walking across the room to sit in a chair—a result you produce from a thought like, "I'd like to sit down," which creates a feeling of desire, which then propels you into the actions of walking and sitting.

Feelings are essential to our everyday life. And yet, we complain about having them, we wish they would go away, we get taught from a young age how to stifle them, and sometimes we're willing to do just about anything to avoid feeling them.

Avoiding your feelings

We *all* avoid feelings! Even this many years into my mindset journey, I still occasionally find myself picking up my phone to scroll on social media or wandering over to the pantry to get a snack when instead I could simply feel my emotions. This is not a problem with you personally; it's just biology.

Your brain is hardwired to seek pleasure and avoid pain—this is your most basic survival mechanism, and even though you can override it on a case-by-case basis, it will always be the default. So, let's examine what's going on biologically with your feelings—just like we did with your thoughts in chapter 2—in order to gain some agency over this natural avoidance tendency.

First, you have a thought, which is a spark of electricity in your brain that's informed by every perception you've ever had. Next, that thought creates your feeling, which is the flood of chemicals (hormones) released by your brain in response to the electrical spark of your thought. Those chemicals produce physiological responses in your body, such as clammy skin, the sensation of tightness in your throat or abdomen, tears in your eyes, tingling in your skin, and so on. Once the release of hormones has created physical sensations, they are now internal body perceptions that your brain is taking in and forming thoughts about, and which you sense in much the same way as any other perception you have from outside your body. There's a good chance that your brain will form a thought like, "This doesn't feel good," when it notices your throat constricting or your stomach churning.

You're having a *thought* about your *feeling*. And, boom! This is when your innate desire to seek pleasure and avoid pain kicks in and drives you to the nearest—or most familiar—source of pleasure. This might be eating, or scrolling on your phone, or getting busy with a project, or simply distracting yourself with other thoughts.

Feeling your feelings instead of lingering in them

Maybe avoidance isn't your issue. For many of us—and I put myself in this category, too—the problem is that we seem to feel everything, all the time. There's a difference between allowing yourself to feel your feelings all the way through, versus thinking more thoughts about them, which results in *lingering feelings*.

When my sister died, I knew that I felt sad. But usually, when I would notice the sad feeling, I would simply continue to think more thoughts, along the lines of, "I just miss her so much, I wish she was still here, and this sucks that I have to deal with our mom all by myself now," and the sad feeling would linger. Sometimes I'd feel sad for most of the day, especially immediately after her passing. One day about six months after she died, I walked back into my house after a run and I had a flash of memory of Vicki out of the blue that absolutely gutted me. I sat down in my desk chair and started sobbing. Not just regular crying, but a deep, gut-wrenching wail that could have come from a wild animal. And while I was crying, I asked myself a question that changed my entire life. I had noticed that my body was churning and heaving and felt like it was turning itself inside out, so I wondered, "Am I going to throw up?" With those six simple words, my brain shifted from thinking more *thoughts* to actually paying attention to the *feelings inside my body*.

I turned my focus to my stomach first, to determine whether or not I needed to find an appropriate receptacle for impending vomit. As it turned out, I was not feeling nauseous, even though my stomach seemed tightly clenched. My heart, throat, and chest felt constricted, and even my hands were squeezed into fists. Though I could still breathe, my lungs felt like they were on fire. I had the very real sensation of falling into a bottomless pit, as though my organs were reacting to elevated g-forces. I was sweating profusely. My heart was pounding loudly in my ears, and there was a tingling, almost itchy feeling in the palms of my hands.

I was able to notice all of these sensations and more, purely from the "good luck" of wondering if my stomach was betraying me. That one question paved the way to recognizing my feelings as a function of my *body* rather than my brain.

Why this is important

The modern human brain has around sixty thousand thoughts a day, which is approximately forty-two thoughts every minute. And of those, scientists suspect that around 90 percent are repetitive—if you've ever had a song stuck in your head, you know this to be true. Between this biology and our socially reinforced reluctance to express emotions, it's no wonder that we create lingering feelings for ourselves. But feelings are meant to be temporary.

Remember that for every hormone that starts a reaction, there's another one to stop it (see page 46 for a refresher). That's exactly what happens with your feelings, too! The physiological symptoms of feelings that you feel in your body are from hormones, which are "started" into your bloodstream because of the spark of electricity of your thought, and that will do their job (which is to spur you into action), and then be "stopped" by another hormone.

When I was in the middle of feeling that deep grief for my sister and asking myself about my stomach, lungs, and strangely itchy palms, there was a brief moment when I worried that I would feel this way forever, that because I had started crying, I would never stop. Thankfully, in that same moment, I also noticed that my breathing felt different—less labored and jagged, though still not quite my regular rhythm. Again, this was a stroke of luck, because it kept me in the moment rather than off on a train of worried thoughts about how I wouldn't be able to function if I was going to cry for the rest of my life.

Instead of going back to my brain, I stayed in my body, and soon the sensations started to dissipate. And then they were gone completely. Nobody was more surprised than I was about this. My heart rate returned to normal, my breathing slowed, my stomach and chest and fists unclenched, my tears stopped, and my skin lost its clamminess. For the first time in my long, emotional life, I had felt a feeling all the way through.

How to Feel Your Feelings in Four Simple Steps (IDEA)

1. **Identify** that you're having a feeling. This might seem obvious, but sometimes it's really not! When you're in the thick of it—especially if you were socialized to manage your feelings by stuffing them down or are so used to reacting first and analyzing later—it can be difficult to notice that you're having one.

2. **Describe** or narrate the physical sensations. Much like allowing yourself to journal completely uncensored, don't overthink this part of the process as though you need to get it right. Whatever words come to you are getting the job done. Personally, I notice that I come up with a lot of clichés—my stomach is in knots, or I'm seeing red, for example. This isn't a test, and there are no extra points for more descriptive language. In my own practice of feeling my feelings, I've developed a checklist of questions to ask myself, with the desired result being that I've noticed and described as many aspects of the feeling as possible. For example: Where do I feel it the most in my body—head, throat, chest, stomach, or limbs? Does it have a color, shape, or smell? What adjectives would I use to describe it—sharp, tight, bubbly,

heavy? Is it moving or staying in the same place? Does it have a texture? Does it seem solid, liquid, or gaseous? After I've gone through the checklist once, I do it again, to see if the feeling is changing in any way. It usually is, as the "stop" hormones are being released and the "start" hormones are being chased out of my bloodstream. Over the years of feeling my own feelings and coaching my clients through feeling theirs, I've discovered that every feeling has its own unique sensations, and if you can stay curious and attentive to them, it's actually fun to find new words to describe each one.

3. **Express** yourself safely. As we've learned, your feelings are supposed to propel you into action, but sometimes those actions aren't in your best interests. We've all shouted at somebody we love and then regretted it or felt ourselves starting to cry during a meeting with our boss. The trick is to lovingly refrain from doing some of the less-convenient physical actions your feelings are trying to drive while still noticing and describing the sensations in your body. If it's safe for you to cry, shout, or laugh, then help yourself! But remember that those actions are a distraction from noticing the physical sensations inside of you, and don't get carried away. Punching a pillow doesn't actually relieve your anger, but paying attention to the "jumpy" vibrations in your torso and limbs that make you *want* to punch a pillow will.

4. **Allow** the feeling to exist in your body. Most feelings will dissipate on their own in about 90 seconds, but some will go away quicker, and some will take longer—presumably due to the specific hormonal cocktail your particular thought unleashed. No matter how long it takes, continue to notice, describe, and express yourself safely.

Describing Your Feelings without Language

As you might expect, I'm a very "language-centric" thinker. So, my development of this IDEA process to feel your feelings all the way through includes describing your feelings in words, but that is not the only method available to you. I have worked with clients who feel their feelings with art, geometric math, and movement to embody their feelings, and these options—or any other that you feel drawn to—are available to you, too. If there is a medium that your brain understands as innately as language, feel free to use it—with the caveat that you should also beware of trying to dissipate the feelings by "getting them out of you" onto paper or into movement. The most important aspect of feeling your feelings is allowing them to exist in your body and dissipate on their own.

Why You Should Feel Your Feelings

The biggest benefit of feeling your feelings all the way through is that it will help you recognize your thoughts as thoughts. Here's the thing about journaling: No matter how much you slow this process down to examine one single thought at a time, you are still having nearly a thought a second, and many of those thoughts will be about your thoughts and about the feelings your thoughts are creating rather than the thoughts you're trying to focus on.

We can see this in action using the Two-Step Tool, going back to the previous example (all the way on page 88, about changing my exercise routine). When I wrote the sentence "This shouldn't be happening to me," tears sprang to my eyes immediately, which sparked an avalanche of other thoughts unrelated to the journaling prompt—*I don't want to cry right now, Who knew I felt this angry?, I hate crying, I have to get through this list, Stop crying, You're such an idiot, You don't have time for this, Why is this making me cry?*—and distracted me from the task at hand.

Could I have buckled down, refocused, and continued on? Sure. But those thoughts about my feelings would still have been bubbling in the background, making this work harder than it needed to be. By feeling your feeling and allowing it to dissipate naturally, you are getting it out of your system, and making room for other feelings.

When journaling with the Two-Step Tool, remember that you need to have space for the feeling of compassion, in order to look at your thoughts and feelings and gain self-awareness. Now, having felt my feeling, I was ready to continue, by putting the phrase "I think" in front of each sentence.

I think I don't want to.

I think I hate that my body is different now.

I think I wish I could stay the same.

I think I don't want to change.

I think I don't know what to do.

I think I hate this different body.

I think menopause sucks.

I think I don't want to.

I think I have to be so careful about everything now.

I think I don't want to think so hard.

I think I like my routine the way it is.

I think I want to keep doing what I've been doing.

I think this shouldn't be happening to me.

Feeling the feeling all the way through released the pain, prevented the feeling from lingering, and opened the door to compassionately observing that the thought "This shouldn't be happening to me" (notice that it's not even in all caps anymore) is a *thought*. And now it's time to take a look at what feeling each of these thoughts create.

I think I don't want to. [Bad/Petulant]

I think I hate that my body is different now. [Bad/Angry]

I think I wish I could stay the same. [Bad/Wistful/Sad]

I think I don't want to change. [Bad/Petulant]

I think I don't know what to do. [Bad/Helpless]

I think I hate this different body. [Bad/Angry]

I think menopause sucks. [Bad/Annoyed]

I think I don't want to. [Bad/Petulant]

I think I have to be so careful about everything now. [Bad/Pressured/Restricted]

I think I don't want to think so hard. [Bad/Petulant]

I think I like my routine the way it is. [Bad/Whiny]

I think I want to keep doing what I've been doing. [Bad/Petulant]

I think this shouldn't be happening to me. [Bad/Powerless]

And, finally, let's label these thoughts as being either HELPFUL or UNHELPFUL by writing the appropriate word next to each sentence and taking a moment to allow our brain time to recategorize each of them individually.

I think I don't want to. [Bad/Petulant] UNHELPFUL

I think I hate that my body is different now. [Bad/Angry] UNHELPFUL

I think I wish I could stay the same. [Bad/Wistful/Sad] UNHELPFUL

I think I don't want to change. [Bad/Petulant] UNHELPFUL

I think I don't know what to do. [Bad/Helpless] UNHELPFUL

I think I hate this different body. [Bad/Angry] UNHELPFUL

I think menopause sucks. [Bad/Annoyed] UNHELPFUL

I think I don't want to. [Bad/Petulant] UNHELPFUL

I think I have to be so careful about everything now. [Bad/
Pressured/Restricted] UNHELPFUL

I think I don't want to think so hard. [Bad/Petulant] UNHELPFUL

I think I like my routine the way it is. [Bad/Whiny] UNHELPFUL

I think I want to keep doing what I've been doing. [Bad/Petulant]
UNHELPFUL

I think this shouldn't be happening to me. [Bad/Abject
Powerlessness] UNHELPFUL

What if you don't know how to feel your feelings?

Sparks of thoughts and floods of chemicals are all well and good, but
what if . . . well, what if you don't seem to experience feelings like
that? I know I've made it sound as though feeling your feelings is the
most natural and easy thing in the world. And technically, it *is* natural, but that doesn't make it easy. In fact, for many women, finding
feelings inside your body is incredibly difficult, and here's why.

- You were socialized to ignore or override your body's signals
  from very early childhood—only being allowed to eat or play
  or go to the bathroom at certain times of the school day—well
  into adulthood, where you've almost certainly had a job that
  demanded ignoring your body in favor of accomplishing a task.

- You learned to accommodate pain or discomfort for a variety
  of reasons, up to and including fashion (I'm looking at you,

pointy-toed, high-heeled shoes!), childbirth, digestive issues, or autoimmune diseases.

- You were taught, either overtly or by example, to control your emotions by shoving them down, pretending they didn't exist, or avoiding them altogether.

- You slowly stopped paying attention to your body because of your brain's innate desire to seek pleasure and avoid pain— when the pain in this scenario was the discomfort of existing in your body as it gained weight or lost fitness, your only option was to disconnect from it.

- You were taught to value thinking (which for many of us was equated to our intelligence, and even our personal worth) over feeling (which was likely positioned as "foolish" or "impractical").

No matter the underlying reason, the current result is that when you are guided to "just look inside your body to find your feelings," you're left wondering what the heck I'm talking about.

Your brain has superpowers, and so does your body

Not to fear because you have yet another superpower, and this one connects your brain with your body! Interoception—like metacognition and neuroplasticity—is a skill you were born with and have likely never been taught how to use. Just like your brain's other superpowers, the way to unlock this one is through simple practice. And, of course, it means that you'll need to be on board with feeling awkward and thinking that you're never going to be good at it, because that's the path to mastering any skill. **Interoception is your brain's ability to sense and communicate what's going on inside your body—it's the ability to know how you feel.**

You might be thinking, "Pahla, I just told you I don't know how to feel!" and yet, here I am, insisting that you do. Before you put the book down in frustration, let me clarify that you might not currently know how to feel your feelings in your body, but that you do have the ability to *learn*. Interoception has two parts, sensing and communicating. There's a very good chance that your brain and body have simply stopped communicating with each other. It's not that the feelings aren't there, it's that you've stopped receiving the signals. I like to imagine this like a radio. Even when it's turned off, or tuned to a different station, the signal from the station you want is still being broadcast—you just have to turn the knob to find it.

Your Turn: Practice Feeling Feelings in Your Body

One of my favorite self-awareness tricks is to pretend that whatever I'd like to develop self-awareness about is happening to somebody else. It sounds counterintuitive—you would think that if you want to be aware of yourself, you should be thinking about yourself! But sometimes all that *thinking about yourself* feels like pressure, as though there's a right and wrong way to go about it. So, to ease that pressure, I like to ask myself how I think somebody else (who is definitely not me, of course) would accomplish the thing.

When it comes to feeling feelings in your body that you're not entirely sure you are capable of feeling, try asking, "What do I think anger feels like in somebody else's body?" Phrased in this way, you can think of it as an intellectual puzzle, instead of a test that you could pass or fail. From this place of curiosity, you might decide that the feeling probably includes an elevated heart rate, because you've noticed that people sometimes get red in the face. (Your observations will be based on how other people look and act when they're reporting a feeling of anger.) They might feel tension in their neck, shoulders, or hands, because sometimes veins there become more visible or the person clenches their fists. Also, you've observed that sometimes people's voices change when they're angry, so there might be a sensation of tightness in their throat or down in their chest and lungs. And you've noticed that people seem to have trouble seeing or hearing—or at the very least, they don't seem to listen to reason, so you suspect that their heads might feel "fuzzy." Finally, we've all heard the cliche about "seeing red" when you're angry, so maybe there's something to that, too.

These are great observations, and an excellent starting place for looking for your own feelings. By very slowly using these points like a checklist, you can begin to develop your own sense of what this feeling could feel like in your body. Note that the difficulty increases as you go down the list, so don't worry if you can't do them all—or even any of them—the first time you try.

- Close your eyes and see if you can become aware of your heartbeat. You can place your index and middle finger gently on your neck or wrist. Would you describe your heartbeat as fast, or slow, or something in between? Are there any other words that simply pop into your head? (Remember, there's no wrong answer here—the Two-Step Tool is all about listening to both your brain and your body without judgment.)

- Squeeze your hands into fists and pay attention to what your fingers and palms feel like. Do you notice the tension? See if you can imitate tension like that in your neck or shoulders, but be careful not to squeeze too hard and hurt yourself. Can you think of a time when you've felt tension like this before? Do you think you were angry?

- Can you create a feeling of tightness in your chest or throat? Don't worry if you can't do this on command—can you remember a time when you noticed your throat or chest feeling constricted?

- What do you suppose "fuzzy" would feel like in your head? Have you ever felt such a thing, like when you woke up suddenly in the middle of the night? How do you suppose that might be different if you were angry?

- What do you think it would actually look like to "see red?" Have you ever been in a situation where something like this has happened to you?

How Your Feelings Help Your Fitness

Practicing your interoception also helps you build muscle, increase bone density, improve your cardiovascular system, lose weight, and—you guessed it—love your body. You may be wondering how all of these are related. Here's how it works: First, you learn to become aware of the inner workings of your body by noticing your heart rate, your sweat, or tension in certain muscles. Next, you learn to describe those sensations, which broadens your awareness. Then, after you've been practicing in a controlled setting, you will naturally begin to notice your body in other situations, too—particularly while you are exercising. Because of this awareness, you will recruit your muscles more effectively and efficiently during your workouts, and your stronger muscles will send positive feedback to your brain, which in turn helps you notice and develop them even more. Next, your stronger body will elicit thoughts of admiration and wonder, which create loving feelings that you can now *feel* in your amazing body. Learning to feel your feelings will teach you how to love your body.

Borrow This (Possibly) Helpful Thought

As (possibly) helpful thoughts go, this is one of my absolute favorites: **My body is a miracle.**

I love this one so much! It honestly makes me giddy every time I say it to myself because it's so true (even though, of course, it's a thought). My brain has no trouble at all finding ample evidence of why I believe it—right this very minute, your body is performing billions of undetectable processes like filtering toxins out of your blood and turning food into energy that will keep you alive several months or even years from now, while you're sitting on your couch reading a book written in a language that somebody with a brain like yours simply made up out of thin air! I mean, *come on.*

Also, I love this (possibly) helpful thought because it says absolutely nothing about the way my body looks, what it can do, or even how it feels today. I find it helpful because it's both specific (*my* body) and broad (*a miracle*) and describes every living thing on Earth. For me, this sentence evokes a feeling of *wonderment*, which is right up there with calm certainty on my "Favorite Feelings" list.

But, of course, this thought is only helpful for you if it feels good to you. So, put your feelings practice to use and tune in with your body. How do you feel when you think "My body is a miracle"— relaxed? Agitated? Disbelieving? If you feel good, it's helpful, and if you feel bad it's unhelpful.

Everything We Learned in This Chapter

~

- You are not going to spontaneously love your body just because you've lost weight, but you can create loving feelings about your body on purpose by thinking loving thoughts.

- Menopause has changed your health risks, and now that estrogen isn't protecting your heart, bones, and muscles, it's up to you to change how you work out.

- A well-rounded menopausal exercise routine includes adequate cardio, regular strength training, and daily balance practice.

- Even without estrogen, your body can and will adapt to consistent exercise, which can improve your heart health, increase your bone density, and strengthen your muscle tone.

- You probably have some Really Unhelpful Thoughts about your changing menopausal body, which create painful or uncomfortable feelings.

- Feelings are involuntary physiological reactions to hormones in your bloodstream, which were sparked by the neuroelectric impulse of your thought. These responses are completely normal, meant to convey information and spur you into action, and designed to be felt temporarily.

- Sometimes we resist or avoid feeling our feelings, but the best course of action is simply to think of feelings as IDEAs— Identify, Describe, Express, and Allow.

- You might currently struggle to feel feelings in your body, but you have the superpower of interoception, which you can learn to harness.

- Practicing interoception can lead to both fitness and mental health gains.

CHAPTER 6

How to Stop Dieting and Start Listening to Your Body

How to Stop Dieting

Imagine where you'll be in a few years: You're at your goal weight, feeling comfortable in your skin and confident about your food choices. You're not feeling angsty or living with "diet thinking"—you know, how you used to be constantly worried about eating too much or eating the wrong thing. Maintaining your weight isn't something you spend much time thinking about, it's just a collection of sustainable habits that you've picked up over the years. It feels natural and healthy to be this weight. You're eating an amount of food that feels really good in your body. You're never stuffed and uncomfortable, and you are only hungry when it's time to eat. You're also eating a nice mix of foods that are healthy for you and give you energy, as well as enjoying treats, and it all feels amazing. This is pretty different from your thoughts and feelings right now.

Here's something you need to know: **Losing weight won't magically stop you from thinking "diet" thoughts.** You know the ones I'm talking about—the nagging voice that doesn't let you just enjoy a slice of pizza, or the cold feeling of dread when you're about to step on the scale (even when you've been easily maintaining your weight for months or even years). That efficient brain of yours has had years of practice judging your food choices and worrying about the numbers, and that doesn't just go away when you reach your goal weight.

The 5-0 Method Advice: You Can Eat Anything

Before we go any further, let me share some counterintuitive advice that will set you free from everything you've heard in the past about what you "have to do" to lose or maintain your weight: **Eat the foods you already enjoy in portion sizes that make sense for your goals, while paying attention to how the food feels in your body.**

You can eat dessert, you can eat potato chips, you can drink wine, you can go out to eat, or you can grab some fast food on your way home from work. Nothing is off-limits. The "catch" is that you'll want to log your calories before you eat, so you can hit your target for the day, and you'll make notes after you eat, so your body can give you information about how the food feels. This advice isn't a license to eat *as much* as you want, it's permission to eat *the things* you want, while learning how to make choices that your body enjoys as much as your brain.

Here's why this works: You think about sixty thousand thoughts a day, and according to some experts, up to 90 percent of those thoughts are repetitive—what I've referred to as automatic or efficient thoughts. Now imagine that one day you decide to change everything you're eating. Different breakfast, different lunch, different dinner, all new snacks and beverages—the whole shebang. You've already seen how uncomfortable it is to challenge just one thought at a time, can you picture challenging *thousands* of them, every day?

You would lose your mind!

And yet, you've probably done this exact thing before, haven't you? I mean . . . haven't we *all*? Every time I started a new diet, I would throw out everything I liked to eat—thinking that it must be the food itself that was making me gain weight rather than the portions I was eating—and start in with "healthy stuff" so I could meet my goals. Some of those diets lasted a few days or weeks, but almost none of the food choices have stood the true test of time.

My advice? Baby steps. Your brain *loves* baby steps! Let me be very clear that you're never "tricking" your brain into doing anything, you are simply working within its chosen parameters. When you work with your brain, instead of against it, you can accomplish amazing things. Your brain values efficiency above nearly everything else, so it simply won't tolerate large-scale changes. This means your best bet for success is to start with the foods you already eat, and work on portion sizes first. Getting your portion sizes in line to meet your caloric target means that you can have some (relatively) quick success with weight loss, while making only minimal changes to your daily habits. Your efficient brain will like this and probably not cause you too much discomfort. If you are currently eating significantly over or under your calorie target, you won't want to jump directly to your target; instead move toward it slowly. The larger the changes, the more uncomfortable you'll be—which of course increases the likelihood of quitting altogether, as your brain seeks pleasure and avoids this discomfort.

In order to stop dieting, we're going to explore where and how you acquired your pervasive automatic thoughts about how to eat for weight loss, the actual science behind "healthy" foods, and then, of course, we'll apply the Two-Step Tool to your thoughts to decide which ones you want to keep and which ones are getting kicked to the curb.

Is a Calorie Really Just a Calorie?

One of the misconceptions I hear frequently when people repeat my own advice back to me about eating the foods you love in portions that make sense while paying attention to how they feel is that I'm saying "a calorie is a calorie," and that's why you can eat anything. Not only is this untrue, but it's not why I give this advice. Your body will lose weight when you eat the *right number* of calories, and my recommendation is that, over time, you find the *right type* of calories to suit your personal needs.

An apple calorie is definitely not the same as a Doritos calorie. And neither of those is the same as a yogurt calorie or a chicken breast calorie! All foods are their own unique combination of calories, carbs, proteins, fats, vitamins, and minerals and will therefore feel and react differently in your body—combined with the complex emotional connections we make with certain foods. This is why I don't make specific suggestions about what you should eat other than to empower you to know what feels good to *you* both physically and emotionally.

Your body will feel its most energetic and run its processes with the best efficiency on healthy, nutrient-dense foods, eaten in an appropriate quantity, but shaming yourself into eating that way will feel terrible. Finding the exact right balance of eating foods that run your body well and feel good emotionally is a balancing act that only *you* can figure out.

Where "Diet Culture" Comes From

The first time I went on a diet, I was nine years old. My young brain had already absorbed enough messages about dieting and weight loss to offer me numerous automatic thoughts about my weight.

And further, my brain was prepared to solve the "problem" of my weight with the solution it had seen countless times at home and in the media: by restricting how much I was eating and avoiding foods I enjoyed because they were fattening. Goodbye, afternoon snack of cookies, and hello, hunger pangs.

I spent the next thirty-odd years in a constant mental state of *dieting*, whether I was heavier or thinner or in between. Those persistent automatic thoughts—about what I could and couldn't eat, and how much, and when, and why, and what it would do to my body composition—stayed with me no matter what the scale said. And now that I understand how brains work—specifically, that they value efficiency above all else—I get why losing weight or being at my goal weight didn't magically change my mind about how and what I was "allowed" to eat.

In the same way that you have taken in billions of perceptions, categorized them, created a thought to explain what you've perceived, and then—when that thought wasn't challenged—repeated it to yourself to form a neural pathway, and now continue to find evidence for its truthfulness every time you butt up against it, so too has every other person on the planet. (See chapter 2 for a thorough explanation of this process, page 56.) Over time, with hundreds of unchallenged thoughts running around, being represented in the media, and passed verbally among family and friends, we as a society have developed certain ideas and behaviors we call *cultural norms*. There are plenty of examples of how normalizing behavior as a society is for the greater good—not condoning cannibalism comes to mind immediately—and just as many that could be considered unhelpful, such as the so-called *diet culture* we live in today.

The desire for thinness and ubiquitous conversation about dieting to attain a certain weight standard in our culture is neither bad nor good. They are simply a collection of repetitive, unmanaged thoughts, shared by a large number of people, that have become a cultural norm. If you want to, you can absolutely challenge these thoughts, and that's what we're doing in this chapter.

The problem with *diet thinking*

Technically, there's nothing wrong with the word *diet* or so-called diet thinking, because one definition of the word *diet* attributed to the Oxford English Dictionary is quite banal: "the kinds of food that a person, animal, or community habitually eats." And, in truth, it's good for your health and well-being to think about what you're eating and plan strategically for what you will eat in the near future to maintain your good health. You will—again, according to the dictionary—be on a *diet* your whole life.

The real issue for most of us lies in further definitions of diet, which explicitly use the words *restrict* and *restriction* as verbs. You and I both know that when you think you're on a diet, restriction is a *feeling*. And for so long in your life—maybe right up until this moment when I'm pointing it out to you—you've thought that the feeling of restriction was the inevitable byproduct of eating a certain way to lose weight, or counting your calories, or not eating a second helping of your favorite dessert. But as we've learned throughout this entire book, your feelings don't come from the things you *do* at all. Your feelings come from your *thoughts*.

So, what does this mean for you? Well, first of all, if your feelings don't come from what or how much you're eating, then you can eat in any manner you choose—"restrictive" or not—and feel amazing about it, simply because you are thinking amazing thoughts that create amazing feelings. Second, if you've already lost your weight and those "restrictive feeling" thoughts have persisted, you now have the tools—the Two-Step Tool, in fact—to find them in your journal and label them UNHELPFUL.

Unpacking your unhelpful diet thoughts is no small feat. You have been absorbing messages about food from your family, friends, media, and random strangers since the moment you were born. Let me assure you that you never need to untangle this entire ball of yarn, and that often pulling on just a few threads can untie you completely from your dieting mindset.

The interesting truth about food and nutrition science

As compared to the sciences of astronomy or math—which have been around since at least 3000 BCE—the disciplines of food science and nutrition science are relatively young, having been formally studied only within the last century or so. Before it became a field of its own, nutrition was mainly under the purview of chemistry, where scientists discovered the three macronutrients (carbohydrate, protein, and fat) and had a rudimentary understanding of how different foods give us nutritional energy (calories). The first vitamin wasn't even discovered until 1926, and the term *nutrition science* didn't exist until the 1950s.

Complicating matters with nutrition science is the fact that food itself is constantly changing. For centuries, humans have been selectively breeding plants and animals to produce specific qualities that we deem more edible or more convenient (think seedless watermelons). There are very few foods on the market today that are unchanged from the time of your great-grandparents. And with the advent of genetic modification in the 1990s, we opened up a whole new world of possibilities where food is concerned by significantly speeding up the selective breeding process.

Then there's the magnitude of items to study. The food you consume comes from three sources: plants, animals, and chemistry. And from those ingredients, humans have managed to create hundreds of thousands—probably millions—of different dishes. It's no stretch to say that the field of nutrition science is—in number of items to study, if not in size—as vast as astronomy. With the constantly changing landscape of food production, and the sheer volume of combinations available to study, it's safe to say that there's more about nutrition that we don't know than that we do.

To complicate things further, not only are food and nutrition sciences dynamic and ever-evolving fields, but your body is, too. Your body is a walking, talking, thinking, blinking miracle. It's also an experiment of one when it comes to your unique combination of nutrition, digestion, and gastrointestinal "stuff." Your personal biology—which is a product of the specific environment in which you were raised, as well as a long history of adaptations made by your ancestors—interacts with the foods you eat in ways that are unique to you. In addition to the vast array of foods and combinations of how and when you might eat them, there's also the fact that you are host to about one hundred trillion bacteria—known collectively as your gut microbiota—that live in your intestines and affect the way you digest food and gain energy from it.

You acquired these bacteria in your first year or two after birth, and you have been affected by them your whole life. Your gut microbiota is highly individualized, adapts and changes frequently (possibly as quickly as every day or every few days), and is subject to your changing personal environmental factors—such as what you've recently eaten, your stress level, the medications you're taking, and more. And in return, your gut microbiota impacts your immune system, your metabolism, your moods, and your susceptibility to certain diseases.

Oh yes, and menopause is probably affecting your digestion, too. There is much more to learn about how menopause affects your gut microbiota, but the current body of knowledge suggests that declining estrogen may play a role in reducing the diversity of bacteria (which is linked to both obesity and diabetes), and the possibility of permeability in the gut barrier (a controversial condition known as "leaky gut syndrome," which may be associated with varying symptoms of gastrointestinal distress).

I mention all of this to make one point: **You are the authority on your own body.** Yes, there's a good chance that eating a variety of foods from each of the food groups will run your body just fine and feel good emotionally and physically. Rather than blindly accepting expert advice—even mine!—I highly recommend that you examine your thoughts (what we're going to do next) and listen to your body (the second half of this chapter), so that you can empower yourself to make your own best decisions. That doesn't mean not to seek expert advice if you have physical or medical issues that necessitate intervention—you definitely should.

Food Thoughts: "Good" Foods versus "Bad" Foods

We are all judgy. We don't only judge ourselves and other people; we judge *everything*. Haircuts, pets, styles of parenting, the color of the sky during tonight's sunset, and—definitely, absolutely, all day, every day—the foods we're eating and not eating. Because, boy oh boy, does your brain have opinions about food! Some foods are good for you, some foods are bad. Some are healthy, some are unhealthy. Some will help you lose weight, and some won't. Carbs and flour and sugar are the reason you can't lose weight. Protein is the answer to everything. Grains give you belly fat. The real key is to pay attention to fiber. Bananas have too much sugar. Avocados are a good fat.

You are inundated with nutrition advice from dozens of different sources—including social media, newspapers and magazines, the internet, your doctor, your next-door neighbor, and even the labels on the foods you buy at the grocery store. Even right here in this book, I'm offering you my advice, too.

How do you know who's right? Well . . . nobody is. It's up to you to decide how you want to eat. So, let's look at some of these thoughts that you've picked up along the way, and see if they're getting you where you want to go.

You have Really Unhelpful Thoughts (RUTs) about "good" and "bad" food

It's time to get creative with the Two-Step Tool—because it's actually quite versatile once you get the hang of it—and find some of the RUTs you have about food. Rather than asking yourself, "What do I think about food?" which could lead to hours of journaling, let's make two lists.

> ### Journal Prompt: Which foods are good for weight loss?

Salad is good for weight loss.

Low-calorie dressing is good for weight loss.

Low-fat cheese is good for weight loss.

Air-popped popcorn is good for weight loss.

Low-calorie snacks are good for weight loss.

Chopped raw veggies are good for weight loss.

Low-calorie bread is good for weight loss.

Cottage cheese or low-fat yogurt are good for weight loss.

Protein shakes are good for weight loss.

Zero-calorie drinks are good for weight loss.

> **Journal Prompt: Which foods are
> bad for weight loss?**

Pizza is bad for weight loss.

Hamburgers are bad for weight loss.

Beer is bad for weight loss.

Cake, cupcakes, and ice cream are bad for weight loss.

Cookies are bad for weight loss.

French fries are bad for weight loss.

Fast food is bad for weight loss.

Cheese is bad for weight loss.

Eating at night is bad for weight loss.

Eating breakfast is bad for weight loss.

Do you know that these sentences are all thoughts? Trust me, I know you think they're true! But do you know that they're thoughts? Every single thing on this list is an opinion.

I think salad is good for weight loss.

I think low-calorie dressing is good for weight loss.

I think low-fat cheese is good for weight loss.

I think air-popped popcorn is good for weight loss.

I think low-calorie snacks are good for weight loss.

I think chopped raw veggies are good for weight loss.

I think low-calorie bread is good for weight loss.

I think cottage cheese or low-fat yogurt are good for weight loss.

I think protein shakes are good for weight loss.

I think zero-calorie drinks are good for weight loss.

I think pizza is bad for weight loss.

I think hamburgers are bad for weight loss.

I think beer is bad for weight loss.

I think cake, cupcakes, and ice cream are bad for weight loss.

I think cookies are bad for weight loss.

I think French fries are bad for weight loss.

I think fast food is bad for weight loss.

I think cheese is bad for weight loss.

I think eating at night is bad for weight loss.

I think eating breakfast is bad for weight loss.

In chapters past, we've moved on somewhat quickly to the next step of deciding if these thoughts are helpful, but for right now, we're going to let this be. As we discussed earlier, these thoughts have been reinforced for you at every turn, not just in your own brain but out in the world—members of your family believe these thoughts to be true, strangers on the internet believe them, and even other weight-loss experts have probably handed you these thoughts as though they were unimpeachable truths. For some thoughts, it's mind-blowing enough just to recognize that they're thoughts! Give your brain time to process that and don't feel the need to push yourself through the whole process right away.

Be patient with your brain and pay attention to when you're ready to move on to the next step of deciding if your thoughts are helpful. Similar to how you let your brain recategorize a thought as unhelpful, your brain is working in the background on a timeline that will not be hurried just because you're impatient with it. For some thoughts, you'll be ready quickly, while others will take significantly longer. There have been long-held thoughts that I needed months to process, and I wasn't ready to move on until I was ready to move on. Allow the process to take as long as it needs to.

Food Thoughts: What You've Been Sold

Plenty of your "diet thinking" comes from the commercials you see every day for food and beverages, which are vying for your attention and selling you—not on meeting your physiological need for food but rather on your psychological desires for safety, social connection, and happiness. If you drink this beer, you'll have lots of friends and parties with good times. If you eat at this restaurant, you'll show the world how successful you are. Starting your day with coffee means you have a loving and stable home life with your family. While there are some advertisements that offer you the health benefits of particular foods, by and large the messages center on the lifestyle you'd (allegedly) have with the purchase. Advertising is a multibillion-dollar industry because it works. Consumers are enticed to buy food and beverage products they don't need for physical survival through messages that tap into their desire for emotional survival.

RUTs and BUTs

I was recently watching a television show where it seemed as though every single commercial was about food. I had already finished eating for the day, but I found myself wondering if I was hungry. This isn't usually a problem for me, and I noticed that there was another feeling rattling around inside, too, though I couldn't identify it right away. Finally, the urge to eat was so strong that I grabbed my journal and took a look at what I was thinking that was creating such an intense emotion.

> **Journal Prompt: What do I think about eating the pizza in this advertisement?**

That pizza looks so good.

As soon as I wrote down that one sentence, I understood exactly what was going on and what the "mystery" feeling was that I hadn't been able to identify. This main sentence was the thought that was creating the feeling of desire, and had I only thought it once or twice, that feeling probably wouldn't have been very strong. But what was happening instead was that I was internally arguing with this thought, which brought it back around again and again—creating an urgent desire that felt stronger every time.

Here's what it sounded like in my head.

That pizza looks so good, but I'm done eating for the day.

BUT that pizza looks so good. BUT it's not on today's menu.

BUT that pizza looks so good! BUT I don't want to eat more tonight.

BUT that pizza looks so good! BUT I've already had enough today.

BUT that pizza looks so good!

Instead of hearing "That pizza looks so good" just once while the commercial was on, I kept hearing it over and over, even while I was watching the program. Therefore, the feeling of urgency intensified. And the previously unidentified feeling? Oh, that was *guilt*.

BUT thoughts and why you feel guilty

One of the tricks your brain employs to be efficient and use the least amount of energy possible is to agree with itself. In fact, scientists have found evidence that your brain will go out of its way to blatant-ly ignore evidence to the contrary of something it already believes, just so it doesn't have to use more energy. However, when your brain is confronted with two different thoughts and believes them both to be true (a psychological principle known as cognitive dissonance), you are left with a phenomenally uncomfortable feeling—in this case, *guilt*.

Notice that, individually, both sentences create good feelings: "That pizza sure looks good" creates desire, which is a lovely feel-ing, and "I've already had enough today" creates satisfaction, also a wonderful feeling. It's the word "BUT" in between the two sentenc-es that—because they're essentially opposing thoughts—creates the cognitive dissonance that feels terrible.

So, what in the world do you do with these thoughts and that terrible feeling? The same thing we always do—use the Two-Step Tool on 'em!

You'll want to know your stated goal before using the Two-Step Tool (flip back to chapter 1, page 35, for a refresher on stating your goal). This pizza situation is a great example of how this works in real life. You've already examined your thoughts about whether or not pizza is "bad" for weight loss, and you're now aware that that's just a thought. So, there's no imperative here on whether you can or can't have pizza. You can. You have permission from yourself to eat whatever you want. Which means that it's up to you to make an intentional decision to either eat it or not, based on if you have room in your calorie target—rather than acting automatically from the feeling of urgent desire.

In my specific example, I had already met my intake for the day, so my stated goal was easy: I am eating the right amount of calories for my goal. With that stated goal in mind, here's what the finished journal entry looked like, using the Two-Step Tool.

I think that pizza looks so good. [Bad/Urgent desire] UNHELPFUL

I think I'm done eating for the day. [Good/Satisfied] HELPFUL

I think it's not on today's menu. [Good/Decided] HELPFUL

I think I don't want to eat more tonight. [Good/Determined] HELPFUL

I think I've already had enough today. [Good/Satisfied] HELPFUL

Even though I didn't come to my journal to solve a problem, the self-awareness of what I'm thinking and how those thoughts feel can help me make a decision about what to do next. In this case, I chose not to eat pizza.

Just for fun, let's explore a slightly different scenario, so it's clear that you *can* choose pizza, meet your weight-loss goals, and not feel guilty. In this next example, let's say that you're not done eating for the day, you do have calories available, and you're trying to decide what to eat for dinner, but your brain is offering you some automatic thoughts about the pizza.

Journal Prompt: What should I eat for dinner?

That pizza looks so good!

I can't eat pizza.

Pizza's bad for me.

That's way too many calories.

It's fattening.

I have to eat healthy.

I have to be good.

With the stated goal of "I am eating the right amount of calories for my goal," let's first clarify that these are all thoughts.

I think that pizza looks so good!

I think I can't eat pizza.

I think pizza's bad for me.

I think that's way too many calories.

I think it's fattening.

I think I have to eat healthy.

I think I have to be good.

And then identify the feeling each thought creates—again, with the understanding that it's your goal to eat the right amount of calories. Occasionally, at this point in the process, the "truthiness" of some of those old, automatic thoughts start working their magic on you, and you forget why you've come to your journal. You think you want to get away from this uncomfortable feeling and solve your problems. But—even better—you're here in your journal for self-awareness about your thoughts.

I think that pizza looks so good! [True/Good/Desire]

I think I can't eat pizza. [True/Bad/Restricted]

I think pizza's bad for me. [True/Bad/Dejected]

I think that's way too many calories. [True/Bad/Worried]

I think it's fattening. [True/Bad/Worried]

I think I have to eat healthy. [True/Bad/Pressured]

I think I have to be good. [True/Bad/Pressured]

When you are Compassionately Observing this list of thoughts, it's clear why you feel so agitated and uncomfortable—everything feels true, almost none of it feels good, and you just want to eat a bunch of pizza to escape from this discomfort! So, let's come back to your stated goal—"I am eating the right amount of calories for my goal"—and recognize the unhelpful thoughts.

I think that pizza looks so good! [True/Good/Desire] HELPFUL

I think I can't eat pizza. [True/Bad/Restricted] UNHELPFUL

I think pizza's bad for me. [True/Bad/Dejected] UNHELPFUL

I think that's way too many calories. [True/Bad/Worried] UNHELPFUL

I think it's fattening. [True/Bad/Worried] UNHELPFUL

I think I have to eat healthy. [True/Bad/Pressured] UNHELPFUL

I think I have to be good. [True/Bad/Pressured] UNHELPFUL

When you can see your thoughts in black and white, it's easier for your brain to untangle the thoughts from each other. You have one helpful thought—"I think that pizza looks so good!"—and the rest are unhelpful. Once again, even though you don't come to your journal to solve problems or feel better, you now have good information (self-awareness) to help you solve the problem of whether or not to eat pizza. The next order of business is to check the number of calories you have left in your day to make sure pizza will fit, and then *decide intentionally* if you want it. Deciding from a place of self-awareness feels so much calmer and clearer than simply reacting to your automatic thoughts.

Borrow This (Possibly) Helpful Thought

You'll recognize this (possibly) helpful thought from elsewhere in this chapter, but now I'll offer it to you plainly: **I decide what I eat.**

Do you love this? Or did it immediately fill you with self-doubt? For me, this helpful thought—because I definitely find it helpful—reminds me that no matter what kind of behaviors my automatic thoughts and feelings are trying to drive, I have the power to choose. To decide. Speaking of deciding, go ahead and find the feeling this thought creates for you, so you can decide if it's helpful or unhelpful for *you*.

How to Listen to Your Body

So far in this chapter, we've covered the first half of my self-love advice—**eat the foods you already enjoy in portion sizes that make sense for your goals**—and now it's time to tackle the rest of it and put your interoception (see chapter 5) superpower to work—**pay attention to how they feel in your body.** Now we're ready to explore the difference between your feelings and how you feel. For our purposes here—which is to say, the most effective way to help you get to your goal—I'm going to divide your feelings in a way you probably haven't seen before: Hormonal versus Mechanical.

Hormonal Feelings

Hormonal feelings have nothing to do with menopause specifically, but everything to do with how the human body works in general. You have over seventy hormones that are produced in your endocrine glands and act as "chemical messengers" that regulate nearly every process in your body. Your brain receives information from a part of your body that needs something. Say your pancreas sends the message that your blood sugar is low. Your brain tells one of your endocrine glands to produce the hormone that will make that thing happen. In this case, it tells the endocrine gland in your stomach to produce ghrelin (the so-called hunger hormone).

Then the endocrine gland releases that hormone (ghrelin) into your bloodstream, where it travels to whichever part of your body needed a thing (your stomach), and then makes that thing happen (increases gastric acids). When the hormone entered your bloodstream it also delivered the "hunger" message to your brain. You then (probably, unless you've conditioned yourself to ignore it) notice the feeling of hunger in your body, presenting as a growling in your stomach and intestines, as well as the contractions of your stomach muscles known as hunger pangs. This is not meant to be an exhaustive description of this process, nor is it the full picture, because even scientists don't understand everything about how this process works.

Now let's imagine that you've just received a message from one of your employees, telling you that they're quitting, effective immediately, even though they were in the middle of a project that's due by the end of the day. In the blink of an eye, you notice (unless you've trained yourself to ignore it) the feeling of anger in your body, presenting as a pounding heart, a dry mouth, rapid breathing, pressure in your head, and tingling in your arms and legs.

"But, Pahla," you may be thinking right now, "there's no way that hunger and anger are alike. I mean, hunger is . . . *hunger*."

Agreed. But let me also point out how very similar these two processes are and explain why I've lumped them together into this category of hormonal feelings.

Step one of both processes is a *perception*. In the case of hunger, your pancreas sensed the level of sugar in your blood and sent that data to your brain, and in the case of anger, your eyes sensed the contrast of light and dark pixels on an electronic screen and sent that data to your brain.

Step two of both processes is your brain assimilating the data. In the case of hunger, you haven't heard a conscious thought yet, because it didn't need to be processed into language, but there's still a "thought" that spurs the next step. In the case of anger, maybe you heard the thought that's about to send out a hailstorm of hormones or maybe you didn't, but there's a thought there, too.

Step three of both processes is your brain making a decision about what your body needs to stay alive and asking a particular endocrine gland to create the hormones that will do that thing—ghrelin for growling and contractions in the case of hunger, or adrenaline and cortisol for rapid breathing, sweat rate, and heart rate in the case of anger.

Step four is the hailstorm of hormones hitting your bloodstream and doing their thing.

And step five of both processes is you acting on the feelings that are present in your body, by eating something or—this is just a guess—throwing your phone across the room and shouting a swear word. But maybe that's just me?

In both instances, there's a perception, then a thought, then the release of hormones, and then a feeling in your body that drives you to action. Hence, my offering you the category of Hormonal Feelings as one of the ways in which you will pay attention to how your food choices feel.

Is Hunger *Really* a Feeling?

There are plenty of diet coaches who will have you believe that there's a difference between "physical hunger" and "emotional hunger," and I'm going to state for the record that I disagree, for two reasons. First, because physical hunger isn't only physical. It also has an emotional or psychological component—meaning that you can intentionally (or unintentionally, as the case may be) prompt your body to release the hormones that create the sensations of hunger simply by *thinking* about food. Just like your other emotions, your thoughts can create feelings of hunger.

And second, I find the phrase *emotional hunger* to be misleading, because what it's actually referring to is the desire to eat in order to avoid some *other* uncomfortable feeling. So, it's not hunger at all, nor is it likely to share the same physical sensations of growling intestines or stomach contractions. What you might be feeling is stress, sadness, anger, frustration or some other emotion you haven't practiced allowing to exist in your body, and the action you're driven to is the pleasure of eating so you can avoid the pain of that emotion.

"Mechanical" Feelings

You are not a machine, so the word *mechanical* may give the wrong impression. The most appropriate description would be "nervous system," but that sounds too much like an emotion when I am referring to something completely different. "Mechanical" feelings are sensations that you feel inside your body that are created by non-hormonal biological processes. One example would be the feeling of pain, such as that brought on by a sprained ankle. In this section we're going to focus on digestive feelings (because we're paying attention to how your food choices feel in your body), such as bloating, gas, constipation, heartburn, and lethargy. These sensations—like your hormonal feelings—offer you valuable information about what's going on inside your body, but only if you're tuning in and listening to what your feelings are telling you.

When and How to Pay Attention to How Food Feels in Your Body

Now that we have our glossary of terms, let's move on to the skills. Make no mistake, what I'm about to share with you is a skill, just like everything else you've learned in this book. You don't need to be a special type of person to be capable of paying attention to how food feels in your body—you just need to be willing to practice and be kind of lousy at it at first (like we are with all skills).

Before you eat, you'll check in with how you feel hormonally (your hunger), and how you feel emotionally (to gain self-awareness about *why* you're eating).

After you eat, you'll check in with how you feel "mechanically" (what your intestines are doing) to gain self-awareness about *what* you've eaten.

By "check in," of course, I mean that you'll grab your journal, ask yourself a question or a few, and see what your brain and body are telling you. It's the Two-Step Tool!

Some quick notes before we start this practice: First, please notice that we are not checking in hormonally after you eat, because feeling guilty after you've eaten something is not the type of information we are looking for here. Yes, it's worthy of exploring, to decide if those thoughts are helpful (spoiler alert: they're not), but those emotions aren't going to have helpful data upon which you can make future decisions about what to eat. And second, I highly recommend that you start practicing this skill at a time when you aren't hungry or trying to make a decision about what to eat in the immediate future. Remember that you're looking for self-awareness, not to feel better or for help with solving a problem right now. With time and practice this skill will have you feeling absolutely amazing about your choices and will be a wonderful guide for making food decisions! But not yet.

Before you eat: using the Two-Step Tool to check your hormonal feelings

We're going to take a slightly different approach to the Two-Step Tool to gain some self-awareness about why you're eating the foods you've chosen. Remember that the reason we do anything is because of a feeling (feelings drive your actions), so if you're thinking about eating a food—an action—then there's a feeling driving that. Sometimes the feeling is plain and simple hunger—but that's incredibly rare. Most of the time, there are other hormonal feelings about the food itself that are driving your behavior, and that's what you're looking for in your journal—the *feelings* you associate with a particular food.

Be sure you're coming to this work ready to compassionately observe your thoughts and feelings. You're not here to judge yourself, you're here to see what your brain and body have to say about a specific food. Your feelings are information about your *thoughts*, not about who you are as a human being. For this journaling session, I'm sharing an old journal entry about a food I eat occasionally that I associate with great pleasure—my mom's homemade cookies.

The "Before You Eat" check-in consists of two questions, and the first one is looking for only a very simple yes-or-no answer. You'll find this answer in your body, in the form of a rumbling or contracting stomach, as we talked about above. The second question is specifically asking for your feelings—which you'll also find in your body rather than your brain. Start every sentence with the phrase "I feel."

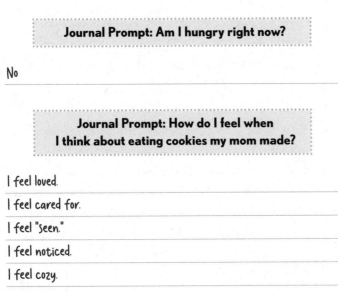

Journal Prompt: Am I hungry right now?

No

**Journal Prompt: How do I feel when
I think about eating cookies my mom made?**

I feel loved.

I feel cared for.

I feel "seen."

I feel noticed.

I feel cozy.

I feel relaxed.

Now, check out this magic. Rather than doing our usual with the Two-Step Tool of trying to find the feeling to decide if these thoughts are helpful—because we already know what the feelings are—the next step is to gently dissociate the feelings from the cookies and remind ourselves that the feeling comes from a thought.

I think I feel loved because of the cookies or my mom, but I feel this way because of my *thoughts.*

I think I feel cared for because of the cookies or my mom, but I feel this way because of my *thoughts.*

I think I feel "seen" because of the cookies or my mom, but I feel this way because of my *thoughts.*

I think I feel noticed because of the cookies or my mom, but I feel this way because of my *thoughts.*

> *I think* I feel cozy because of the cookies or my mom, but I feel
> this way because of my *thoughts.*

> *I think* I feel relaxed because of the cookies or my mom, but I feel
> this way because of my *thoughts.*

So interesting, right? I knew that I loved my mom's cookies, but until I had journaled about them, I didn't understand why they felt so compelling to eat. But now I understand it—my brain thought the cookies were responsible for feelings of love, warmth, relaxation, and connectedness. Of course I'd want to eat them if they were providing me with those feelings! This is fabulous information, but it's only half of our journaling about this topic. Next up is the check-in after eating the cookies.

After you eat: check in with your "mechanical" feelings

I've mentioned that I consider myself more of a Thinker than a Feeler—I'm very comfortable in my head, and when I first started doing mindset work, I took to the whole "find your thoughts" thing like a duck to water. But I'm also an endurance athlete who has struggled mightily to conquer fueling challenges during long races—I'll spare you the gory details, but suffice it to say that I've had my share of GI distress while running—so I've learned how to pay attention to my body, too.

What I'm offering you now is an "After-You-Eat Body Checklist" that I've developed for myself as a person who only feels in tune with my body through my thoughts. If I don't ask myself a specific and direct question about a particular body part that makes it clear what some of my options might be, I often don't notice a feeling in my body. If you have a language-free method of communicating with your innards that works for you, please feel free to use your own.

The point of this check-in is twofold: self-awareness and data gathering. You want to be aware of how your body feels while it is digesting and using the food you've eaten (self-awareness), and eventually you want to use this information to make decisions about eating this food again (data gathering). Thinking about it like a science project might help you observe yourself with compassion, instead of judgment.

Depending on what you've eaten, it can take anywhere from twelve to seventy-two hours for the food to be completely digested and pass through your system. This means that—unless you're only eating one meal a day, which is not my recommendation—it will be difficult to know exactly which food is causing which reaction. Rather than getting bogged down by not knowing the exact cause and effect in your body, simply check in with your mechanical feelings several times a day, and only try to home in on a culprit if you're having a particularly unpleasant response. (And, hopefully it goes without saying, if you're having a severe reaction, seek medical attention immediately.)

Personally, I like to do a brief check-in about an hour after I've eaten a meal to record information about fullness and satiety, which can help me make future decisions about portion size, as well as first thing in the morning and right before I go to bed. When you first start practicing this skill, that might feel like a *lot*, so remember that you can take baby steps. Even checking in once a day or once a week is more information than you currently have.

At the top of the journal entry, I make a quick note about what I ate and how much. This might not be necessary if you have this information logged in your calorie counting app—that's up to you. While I'm writing this down, I take a moment to make sure I feel calm, curious, and compassionate (see chapter 2, page 70, for more on Compassionate Observation). And then I start scanning my body, searching for any information it has for me, ready and willing to record what I notice without judgment. Here's the checklist I go through.

1. General torso check—do I feel hungry, full, or just right?
2. Throat and esophagus—is there tightness or burning, like heartburn?
3. Stomach and middle chest—do I have heartburn or nausea?
4. Belly area from lower ribs to navel—do I feel nausea, fullness, or bloating?
5. Lower intestines—do I have bloating, gas, or a constipated feeling?
6. Overall body—does my energy level seem normal, or do I feel lethargic?

And here's exactly what this journal entry looked like after I'd eaten my mom's cookies.

Five snickerdoodles, mid-afternoon before dinner
1. Slightly full.
2. Nothing noted.
3. Nothing noted.
4. Slightly full.
5. Nothing noted.
6. Energy level is different—simultaneously jittery and lethargic.

What to do with the check-in information

I think of this daily "pay attention to how food feels" check-in as being akin to a combination of your daily journaling and your daily weigh-in—it's information about what's going on with you emo-tionally that you're not trying to fix or change, plus data about your body that can be useful for guiding future decisions. You're not tak-ing notes so that you can change everything up tomorrow. Rather, you're practicing the gentle art of self-love and self-acceptance so that doing so will become a habit. While you're loving and accepting yourself, you *might* also change some of the foods you eat, or the portions in which you eat them.

Many years ago, my eating habits looked very different from how I eat now. Despite my semi-frequent pantry cleanouts and "I'm going to eat nothing but healthy foods!" diets, I still found myself coming back around to comfort foods, mindless snacking, and last-minute, not-so-healthy meal choices. It wasn't until I started taking a com-passionate look at *why* I was eating and how it actually *felt* in my body that I was able to make significant, long-term changes—in tiny baby steps, of course.

So, here's what you're going to do with the check-in information: nothing right away.

Over the course of weeks and months, you might start to notice patterns. If you are handy with a spreadsheet (I'm not), you might enjoy making charts or graphs to see if you can find trends. Allow your brain to work through the information without judgment and be open to the possibility of making changes that feel doable.

It took me months of note-taking to identify what I now call the "too many cookies" feeling I described above in number 6. The feeling wasn't wildly uncomfortable—nor were the cookies a daily habit—so I didn't make the connection right away. When I did find the correlation, that's when I did the "Before You Eat" check-in jour-naling about the cookies. Having the combination of self-awareness and data helped me make a decision about when, how many, and under what conditions I will intentionally choose to eat my mom's cookies: When they're available, I will have a maximum of three, and I will do my best to move other food choices around so that I still meet (rather than exceed) my energy needs for the day.

This brings up one of the most important lessons I can teach you about finding your thoughts and deciding if they're helpful: **Just because you *can* challenge your thoughts—and therefore your feelings, which will therefore change your habits—doesn't mean you *have to*.** There might be foods you eat that aren't serving you nutritionally, but if they're not creating discomfort "mechanically," you can choose to eat them for hormonal reasons. There's no external imperative to make changes in your life.

Doing this hormonal and "mechanical" feelings work was both eye-opening and incredibly empowering for me. For most of my life, I had always felt at the mercy of my food desires. But offering myself the gift of self-awareness led me to make decisions about what I wanted to eat rather than simply going along with the choices my automatic brain handed to me.

Borrow This (Possibly) Helpful Feeling

Wait, you can practice Helpful Feelings, too? Yes, indeed, and this is one of my all-time favorites: **decisiveness.**

When I feel decisive, my shoulders pull back and I stand up straighter. My head feels clear and bright, my stomach is soft, and I can breathe easily. My spine feels strong. Decisive smells metallic (in a good way) and it feels like sunshine. My hips feel balanced and my legs are sturdy. A friend of mine has a feeling she calls "correctly assembled," and I think it must feel very much like *decisive* feels for me. I follow through when I feel decisive, and I don't second-guess myself. I trust my feeling of decisiveness.

What does decisiveness feel like for you? Is it helpful?

Everything We Learned in This Chapter

- Diet thoughts—or the restrictive feelings you have from dieting—are the same as other automatic, efficient thoughts, and getting to your goal weight doesn't eliminate them.

- Instead of dieting, I recommend that you eat the foods you already enjoy in portion sizes that make sense for your goals, while paying attention to how they feel in your body.

- Taking "baby steps" and making incremental changes will lead to sustainable long-term success.

- *Diet culture* is a group of people who share and spread the same automatic, unhelpful thoughts.

- The Two-Step Tool will help you sort through your dieting thoughts and decide if they're helpful.

- You are the expert of your own body.

- Believing that certain foods are "good" or "bad" is a thought.

- The feeling of guilt is the discomfort your brain feels when it's trying to hold two opposing thoughts that it believes are both true.

- Listening to your body is the magic that can help you intentionally decide which foods you want to eat and which foods you don't.

- Interoception (listening to your body) means feeling your emotions as well as noticing your digestive sensations.

- Doing a "Feelings Check-In" before and after you eat is a great way to gather data and build trust with yourself.

- You can decide to eat anything you want.

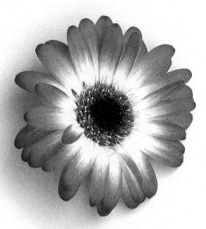

PART FOUR

Embracing Life
After 50

CHAPTER 7

You Can't "Positive Think" Your Way Out of Hot Flashes

Sometimes Menopause Sucks, and That's Okay

Let's call many of the changes that menopause brings your way . . . "fixable." You can definitely lose weight, you can strengthen your bones and muscles, you can protect your heart from cardiovascular disease, you can dismantle your diet thinking and maintain your goal weight for the rest of your life, and—my personal favorites—you can love your body and trust yourself. You can learn new skills, you can find your feelings inside your body, and you can determine which thoughts are leading you to your goal and which ones are stalling you out. You have hidden superpowers you didn't even know about! And those superpowers can help you create anything you want in life . . . unless what you want is to stop having hot flashes and migraines.

We've spent a lot of time in this book accepting that you will feel worse before you can feel better. And now I have some news that you might not want to hear: Sometimes you're just going to feel lousy. Of course, you know that things happen in the world that feel terrible, but is there a little part of you that thinks life would be better if you could just be happy all the time? I suspect that most of us are secretly—or not so secretly—wishing for it. It sounds so nice, so calm, and so pleasant to live in a world where nothing feels sad and you never get angry. But here's the thing you don't realize when you're thinking about this fantasy world. If you didn't feel bad, you also wouldn't feel good.

The reason you notice your feelings at all is because you have so many of them and they all want to propel you to action, but the way you tell them apart is through contrast. In the same way that your brain is always trying to categorize your perceptions by lumping them together, it's also making sure to keep different things separate. You might be thinking, "But I already have plenty of contrast between good and bad in my life—why do I have to have brain fog, insomnia, and vaginal dryness, too?"

Here's why: Because sometimes menopause sucks.

You don't have to make it worse than it is

The real problem with feeling bad isn't the "feeling bad" part—it's wanting so much not to feel bad that you end up feeling worse. When I started gaining menopause weight and learned that women my age take longer to recover from intense exercise, I refused to believe it at first. "Maybe that's how it works for other women, but not me!" I declared defiantly to myself. My body, on the other hand, was like, "Umm, okay. But that's not how this is going to go," and proceeded to march toward menopause as though I didn't have a say in the matter. As it turned out, I didn't have a say in the matter.

Boy, was I steamed about that. "I'll show my body who's boss!" I silently shouted while going out for a long run that I needed significantly longer to recover from than I used to. "This isn't happening," I muttered to myself when I was so stiff and sore it was hard to get out of bed. "It's not supposed to be this way," I whined when the scale went up. Again, it appeared as though my body was the boss. The more I fought against it and the angrier I became, the worse I felt, both hormonally and mechanically. I spent months pushing harder in my workouts in an effort to feel better, with the result that I had constant low-grade injuries and near-total emotional burnout. I was a wreck. Because I wanted to feel good.

This would be a really good story with a happy ending if I could point to a single day where I had a big epiphany—and maybe even a good, long cry—and then I *did* feel better, and everything turned out great. But that's not quite what happened. It turned out that everything I've been telling you so far in this book is true—I made small changes, started doing daily journaling to find my thoughts and decide if they were helpful, and worked on recognizing my feelings inside my body so I could feel them instead of shoving them down. And now, several years into this work, I feel amazing. And lousy.

How to feel lousy in two easy steps

Step one, a thing happens in the world. Step two, you think that thing shouldn't have happened. Maybe—because of all the work we've been doing with finding your thoughts—you recognize that one of those sentences is a thought. (Hint: It's the second one, the one that starts with "You think . . .") But the first sentence isn't a thought. It's reality.

This will sound simple and obvious, but here we go anyway: Reality exists.

And *thinking* that the thing that definitely exists—reality—shouldn't exist is the source of your pain, not reality. Let's clarify with an example: Thinking that you shouldn't be going through menopause—which might sound like, "My body is changing because of menopause, BUT it shouldn't be"—is more painful for you than menopause itself.

We touched on the concept of cognitive dissonance in chapter 6 (in the discussion about guilt, on page 183) and it applies here, too. You are holding two thoughts that are in opposition to one another, and you think they're both true. The difference with this example, though, is that one of them *is* true. You *are* going through menopause (or you've already gone through it, and you're still having these efficient, automatic thoughts that want to fight against it).

When you are choosing between two *thoughts*, the truth is what you decide it is. With our pizza example in the last chapter, "That pizza looks so good" was a thought, and so was "I'm done eating for the day" (see page 182). So, the solution for resolving your dissonance was to simply pick one. When one of your options is reality, though, your choice is clear: Reality is true. But your brain doesn't always want to see it that way.

Here's why it's so easy to get caught up in "This shouldn't be happening" thinking: Remember that your brain is always trying to seek pleasure and avoid pain. Of the two thoughts, "My body is changing because of menopause" is more painful to your brain than "It shouldn't be." Why does your brain think so? Because it's already a step ahead of you and knows what other thoughts you'll think after that initial one. Behind "My body is changing because of menopause" is a cornucopia of automatic, efficient thoughts about how much you don't like change, how much hot flashes suck, and how you're probably going to turn into a dried-up old lady. But when you think "It shouldn't be," your brain gets to go into problem-solving mode. Therefore your brain thinks that "It shouldn't be" is the bee's knees, and it's going to hang on to it for dear life. (Remember from chapter 1 that we've evolved to look for and solve problems! See page 31.)

Then your brain gets caught up in "This shouldn't be happening" thinking because it can't actually solve the problem of something that "shouldn't be" happening when it *is* happening. That's the nature of reality! So around and around your brain goes, searching for a solution that doesn't exist.

Complicating matters further is that the discomfort of cognitive dissonance is itself a *feeling*, which means that it is driving actions, and for many of us those actions are going to be avoidance activities, as when I tried to prove to myself that I wasn't going through menopause by continuing to exercise like I did when I was younger. Your brain tries to escape the feeling of cognitive dissonance, which was created because of your brain trying to escape the feelings of going through menopause.

My advice here is simple and might sound counterintuitive, as it has been throughout this book: **Stop trying to feel better and allow yourself to feel all of your feelings—even the bad ones.**

Advertisers Use Cognitive Dissonance to Sell You Beauty Products

You are getting older, and I can state that with confidence because every single person, plant, and animal on the planet—as well as the planet itself—is getting older with every passing minute. That's how time works. But we also have social norms (particularly in Western societies) that promote youthfulness as the standard for beauty, and there are hundreds of products on the market that exploit your cognitive dissonance about that standard.

You are getting older, BUT youth is beautiful.

In an effort to relieve the discomfort of dissonance, it's your pain-avoiding, pleasure-seeking brain that drives the purchase of lotions, potions, serums, makeup, supplements, and appliances that promise you the glow of a girl in her twenties. But you're not in your twenties anymore, so the cognitive dissonance persists. And of course the answer to that—according to advertisers—is to buy more products!

Why Feeling Worse Will Help You Feel Better

Do you have any idea how much time you spend right now trying to avoid your uncomfortable feelings? According to my smartphone, I spend nearly two hours a day playing games, and another hour and a half on social media—technically, some of that's job related, but still—and I suspect there's at least another hour a day taken up with "busy-work" that I give myself because I'm struggling to accomplish my real work. Writing this book has been eye-opening for me in that respect. So far in writing on this chapter, I've "needed" to do the dishes, check to see if my son is at work or at school, text my husband with something inconsequential, and take the recycling outside to the bin—all because some of the ideas and sentences weren't flowing as easily as I would have preferred. (The irony is not lost on me.) And it's not just a matter of wasting time. Some of us avoid our feelings by spending money, eating food, smoking, drinking, or engaging in other behaviors that we wish we wouldn't, but that still seems preferable to facing our feelings. This is all thanks to our lovely brain, of course, which is always seeking pleasure and avoiding pain.

Are your feelings really painful?

If you've ever broken a bone, sprained a ligament, or accidentally cut your thumb wide open with a really sharp kitchen knife while you were foolishly slicing a tomato toward you instead of using a cutting board (true story), then you have felt physical pain. So, you know what that's like: There's an acute phase when the injury occurs where the pain doesn't even register in your brain because it's so strong and/or unexpected. Then there's the burning, throbbing, stinging, or searing pain that accompanies some sort of first aid or medical intervention. And then—depending on the severity of the injury—you might require pharmaceutical pain relief for a few days while your body begins to repair the damage. When you use the word *pain*, you're usually referring to something physical. Feelings aren't like that *at all*.

The involuntary physiological sensations associated with the release of hormones—what we've been referring to throughout this book as feelings or emotions—are, by their very nature, housed completely inside of you and are short-lived. Their purpose is to get your attention, prepare your body for action, and then compel you to do something quickly, instead of thinking slowly.

When you have a thought—a spark of electricity in your brain—it triggers the release of hormones such as adrenaline and cortisol into your bloodstream that affect different parts of your body and produce symptoms like an elevated heart rate and breathing rate (which increases your sweat rate), elevated blood pressure, and dilated eyes. Depending on what emotion you're feeling, you might notice sensations such as a tingling feeling in your limbs, intestinal distress (when your body rushes blood to your major muscle groups in a "fight or flight" response, it also temporarily shuts down digestion), or a tightness in your throat. The hormones that course through your veins while you're feeling an emotion will only affect your body for about 90 seconds—but only if they're allowed to run their course naturally. Recall from chapter 5 how often we all engage in avoidance of—or lingering in—our feelings (see page 155).

The Net Positive Effect of Feeling Your Negative Feelings

It's a hard sell when I tell you to feel your uncomfortable (but not painful) feelings. So let's explore what you'll gain from them. When you feel your feelings, you will

- save time (as well as possibly money, relationships, and your health),

- increase your confidence and self-trust,
- reduce the difficulty and fear of feeling your feelings in the future, and
- gain agency over your thoughts.

Let's look at each of these benefits in more detail.

Save time, money, relationships, and your health

You know how I spend two hours a day on my phone playing games? A couple of years ago, it was nearly triple that amount. For me, the direct effect of allowing my feelings to exist in my body and dissipate on their own has been increased productivity and creativity, because I'm no longer wasting (as much) time or brain space on avoiding them. For many women, feeling your feelings will reduce stress eating, emotional spending, or constant bickering with your partner. When you are not running away from—or stewing in—your feelings, you will have more time and energy to do what you truly enjoy.

Increase your confidence and self-trust

Asking yourself to do hard things and then doing them is one of the greatest gifts you can possibly give yourself. During the actual feeling of your feelings, you will trust yourself to accomplish the task, and afterward, you'll have evidence that you're capable of doing it. This is the very definition of a virtuous cycle (as opposed to the vicious cycle of thinking that you can't feel your feelings, which leads you to continue avoiding them).

Reduce the difficulty and fear of feeling your feelings in the future

Allowing emotions to exist in your body is a skill, which means that—like any skill—you will get better with practice. Remember the first time you drove a car, how you had to pay attention to every single detail and it all seemed overwhelming? And now you can drive to work and not remember a single thing about getting there, because you were singing along with the radio. Feeling your feelings will *feel* easier, which means that you won't be afraid of feeling more of them.

Gain agency over your thoughts

You have feelings because of your *thoughts*—not because of things that are happening to your body, or that are happening in the world, or because of something that somebody said or did. When you allow your body to feel the feeling all the way through, you will create the space for yourself to compassionately observe your thoughts (and feelings) from a distance instead of being *in* them. (We explored this a bit in chapter 5, see page 157.)

Let's Feel Some Feelings!

If you are relatively new to feeling your feelings all the way through—and you probably are; nobody taught you this in school—you might want to take breaks between the rest of the sections in this chapter. I encourage you to put in the work and feel through your emotions in real time with me, and sometimes that creates a "feelings hangover."

The flood of hormones in your body is strong—your heart will likely pound, your breathing will quicken, your digestion will be disrupted, and your limbs will feel jittery. As your body returns to homeostasis (balance), sometimes there's a feeling of *overcorrection*, where you're exhausted. I've worked with many clients who needed to take a nap after feeling through their feelings. Rather than rushing through and trying to feel everything in one day, try picking one feeling, and come back to the others on different days. Don't worry, you will work through them all, but there's no hurry.

Here's the list, in order, of the emotions we're going to explore next, so you can choose which one you'd like to work through: Anger, Grief, Shame, and Helplessness.

You may find one or more of them particularly difficult to feel all the way through—years of social conditioning and your biological drive to seek pleasure and avoid pain are always at play—and this is completely normal. Remember to come to this work ready to compassionately observe yourself rather than judge your efforts. This is a new skill you're learning, and it will take practice before you master it.

How I Choose When to Feel an Emotion, and Which One to Feel

Let me start by assuring you that there's no "wrong" way to feel your emotions, unless you somehow manage to injure yourself. Nor is there a "right" way to go about this process—though I will share some of what I consider best practices that have worked for me.

When you are journaling with the Two-Step Tool and looking for self-awareness, start by getting physically comfortable—sitting in a cozy chair, wearing clothes that feel good, not being in a rush, and writing in your favorite journaling notebook. I like to use a bright, jewel-toned pen. These rituals help ground me, and they feel like loving habits that I do for myself. This starts me out in a calm manner and reminds me that this work is good for me. Try to be alone and allow yourself at least 10 to 15 minutes of "me time" to explore what's in your brain.

After choosing a question and starting to write, allow anything that's in your brain to come out of your pen. This has taken me some practice—my urge to censor myself was very strong when I first started this work. If this is challenging for you, too, remind yourself that you're simply looking for thoughts. You just want to know what's in your head. You're not trying to feel better or solve a problem. If you're only here out of curiosity, there's no way to lose.

While the words are flowing out, notice the reaction that your body is having to them. This has also taken practice for me to be able to "hear" both my brain and my body at the same time, so don't worry if you need to take time to do this intentionally when you're first starting out. Get your thoughts out first, and then listen for your feelings.

As I'm listening for my feelings, sometimes I just notice them all and label them—meaning that sometimes the Two-Step Tool is "just" journaling. But occasionally, one of the thoughts or one of the feelings will jump out at me. I call it a *full-body zing* because it feels like a bit of an electric shock. When that happens, I know there's more to explore—either more thoughts behind the first one, or a feeling that needs to be felt. When it's more thoughts, I usually hear a big blank wall of "I don't know," which is my brain's defense mechanism against hearing thoughts that might feel painful. And when it's a feeling that needs to be felt, I usually can already feel it welling up inside me, ready to be described, expressed, and allowed. I allow every bit of my journaling practice to unfold organically, and I trust that I will get out of it exactly what I need to for that given moment. But this wasn't always the case!

When I first started, I often struggled to think of a question to ask myself or to get even one sentence on the page. I often walked away from my journal wondering if it was worth my time. At least half of my sessions felt unsatisfying. But the other half of the time, I would find some epiphany, or really grasp that a thought I was having was just a thought. And I kept coming back for more.

You can use the Two-Step Tool as a jumping-off point to find what works best for you. It's like the old adage, *Know the rules so you can break them.* In the following pages I'm going to walk you through a handful of difficult emotions in a way that works for me, and I offer it to you so that you can find your own way to feel your difficult feelings and set yourself free from them.

The following journal prompts use an out-of-order version of the Two-Step Tool, where I intentionally skipped adding "I think" in front of each sentence until after I'd felt the *zing* feeling all the way through.

Anger

I have a long history of avoiding anger, and still catch myself saying things like, "I don't really like to get angry," even though I can and do feel anger all the way through without incident. My brain offers me the thought that I will be out of control when I'm angry—that I will say and do things that I'll later regret. That was certainly true before I realized that I could simply *feel* angry, without reacting to it or expressing it. Anger can exist inside my body, and it will dissipate on its own.

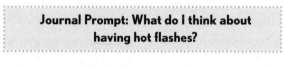

Journal Prompt: What do I think about having hot flashes?

They're annoying. [Bad/Dismissive]

I don't like them. [Bad/Irritated]

They're out of control. [Bad/Out of control]

I HATE THEM. [Bad/RAGE] *Zing*

This feeling erupts inside me like a hot volcano—my head feels like steam is escaping from the top, my face and chest are hot, hot, hot, and my heart is pounding in my ears. I notice that the feeling is not unlike the hot flashes that I'm feeling this rage toward. Am I having a hot flash while being angry at hot flashes? My throat feels tight and I want to cry, but that feels like a misdirect—I'd rather be sad, because that's easier. [When my brain starts thinking about something else in the middle of feeling a feeling, I repeat my question to myself and the answer that created the emotion I want to allow.] What do I think about having hot flashes? I HATE THEM. My hands are clenched. My teeth are clenched. My jaw and shoulders feel tense. I'm breathing heavily. The only thing I can hear is my heartbeat—it sounds annoyingly loud. My stomach feels like it's stabbing me from the inside. My arms are jittery and wild. I can't seem to keep my eyes open, and they're clenched so tightly I actually see red. That's so weird, I thought that was just something people said. My scalp is prickly. I'm drenched in sweat. My legs feel antsy, like I want to run.

My mouth is dry, but my throat isn't as clenched as it was a moment ago. The steam feels like it's almost done. I'm shaky all over and exhausted. My body releases, bit by bit. My hands unclench, my shoulders come down, my jaw loosens. Rage has come and gone.

After the feeling has subsided, it's time to compassionately come back to your journal and remind yourself that this feeling was created from a thought. Not from the fact of hot flashes. Add "I think" in front of each sentence and let it sink in that these are thoughts.

I think they're annoying. [Bad/Dismissive]

I think I don't like them. [Bad/Irritated]

I think they're out of control. [Bad/Out of control]

I think I hate them. [Bad/RAGE]

And then, the gentle and important reminder to your brain that this thought is not helping you feel good about your body, your life, or yourself. Label the thoughts as HELPFUL or UNHELPFUL.

I think they're annoying. [Bad/Dismissive] UNHELPFUL

I think I don't like them. [Bad/Irritated] UNHELPFUL

I think they're out of control. [Bad/Out of control] UNHELPFUL

I think I hate them. [Bad/RAGE] UNHELPFUL

Recognize that hating hot flashes isn't helpful to moving toward my self-love goals, but, simultaneously, if I choose to think that thought, I am capable of feeling the emotion it brings.

Grief

I'd like to say that I'm pretty good at feeling grief because it's the feeling I have the most experience with. And yet, I still resist it sometimes—as we all do. I often think of grief as *inconvenient*, because I know I will cry, which makes my face turn red and my mascara run. I use these as excuses, telling myself I don't have time to be sad right now. But I do. I've practiced grief enough to know that this one's a shooting star for me—bright and hot, but ultimately short-lived.

> **Journal Prompt: What do I think about my hair turning gray and falling out?**

I don't like it. [Bad/Petulant]

I wish I had my old hair. [Bad/Sad]

I'm not the girl I used to be. [Bad/Bereft] *Zing*

The tears are in my eyes before I put the period on the end of that sentence. It's true, it's so true. I'm not that girl and I'll never be her again. I want her back.

These are more thoughts—what's the feeling? Sadness? I'm sad. Grief? I'm *bereft*. My stomach lurches as though I've fallen into a deep chasm. I'm falling, falling, falling. Everything is dark. I can't grab anything, my throat is closing, tears and snot. I'm howling. Everything inside of me is being ripped out, thrown away, my heart is squeezing so tight. I can't breathe. Can I breathe? I can. But it's hard to breathe and it sounds like I'm wheezing, moaning. I can't close my mouth; I want to cry this feeling out of my body. My ears are stuffy, I want to curl up and protect my body but I'm falling, hands out wide, trying to stop myself. [I put my hands on the chair and gently remind myself that I'm safe and I can feel this feeling. I'm not falling, it's a feeling inside my body.] I feel my heart beating hard, my stomach clenching and heaving. It's dark but almost like a tunnel, like there's a little bit of light in front of me. I'm not falling as fast, as wildly.

I can breathe. It's ragged, but it's coming all the way in and filling my lungs. My arms start to relax. I'm not falling. I can see. I need a Kleenex. I lived through grief.

Adding "I think" in front of each sentence brings this thought into sharp focus. Of course this is just a thought. I'm still the girl I always was, and the girl I'll be in the future. I have changed, and I am changing, but I'm always me. I just had a thought.

I think I don't like it. [Bad/Petulant]

I think I wish I had my old hair. [Bad/Sad]

I think I'm not the girl I used to be. [Bad/Bereft]

And of course these thoughts aren't helpful for loving my life and looking forward to my future, so I'll label them as such, and my brain can do its thing.

I think I don't like it. [Bad/Petulant] UNHELPFUL

I think I wish I had my old hair. [Bad/Sad] UNHELPFUL

I think I'm not the girl I used to be. [Bad/Bereft] UNHELPFUL

In place of the grief, I'm left with a deep love for the girl I am. I'm willing to feel my feelings, even when—maybe especially when—they're hard.

Shame

Let me tell you right now that this one is not fun. Shame is a feeling that cuts deep into the core of who you think you are. Other feelings might be about situations that have happened out in the world, but shame is only about you—as though there is something intrinsically wrong with your being, your essence. In my experience, I have rarely heard a thought that created the feeling of shame that sounded like something to actually be ashamed of; rather, it usually comes from something that was important or valuable in your family of origin.

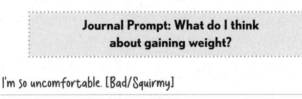

Journal Prompt: What do I think about gaining weight?

I'm so uncomfortable. [Bad/Squirmy]

I'm out of control. [Bad/Defeated]

I don't know what my body is doing anymore. [Bad/Annoyed]

I can't believe this is happening. [Bad/Exasperated]

I'm so stupid. [Bad/SHAME] *Zing*

Hot, hot, hot, hot, hot black coal like a lump, sinking and shrinking inside. Curling in on myself. My heart is pounding and pounding, but slow, dull, sloppy. My lips are shaking, my face is shaking, my eyes are shaking. My arms feel like trees, heavy and wooden. I'm stuck in place. Sunk. Sulfur, stink. I can't see, I can't hear, I'm curling into a ball. My stomach is squeezing tight. I'm disappearing, I'm smoke, smelly. I think I'm crying but I can't tell. My head is squeezing and shrinking, my wooden arms too slow, burning up. Where's my stomach? It's gone. My legs are lead, my hips an anchor, I can't move. Numb. Hot.

I feel the top of my head start to return, gently. Like I was being erased, but now I'm showing up again. Getting clearer and lighter. I hear my heartbeat and it sounds like me. My face still tingles, but I'm breathing and moving my neck and head. I unfurl. Shame didn't burn me down.

After many years of examining this particular thought and feeling this feeling through, I can say with certainty that it *is* a thought.

I think I'm so uncomfortable. [Bad/Squirmy]

I think I'm out of control. [Bad/Defeated]

I think I don't know what my body is doing anymore. [Bad/Annoyed]

I think I can't believe this is happening. [Bad/Exasperated]

I think I'm so stupid. [Bad/SHAME]

And further, these thoughts aren't helpful in my quest to love and respect myself and my beautifully aging and changing body.

I think I'm so uncomfortable. [Bad/Squirmy] UNHELPFUL

I think I'm out of control. [Bad/Defeated] UNHELPFUL

I think I don't know what my body is doing anymore. [Bad/Annoyed] UNHELPFUL

I think I can't believe this is happening. [Bad/Exasperated]
UNHELPFUL

I think I'm so stupid. [Bad/SHAME] UNHELPFUL

After feeling through shame, I'm aware of how good I feel—calm and relaxed, as though I've weathered a difficult storm. This moment of quiet afterward is one of the reasons I've learned to enjoy feeling my uncomfortable feelings.

Powerlessness

When you start feeling your feelings all the way through, you will probably develop your own ranking system for them the way I have with mine. For me, powerlessness gets a zero out of ten stars, do not recommend. And here's why: for a long time, I associated this feeling—which is to say that I was resisting feeling it—with *being* powerless. This feeling is vulnerable and raw, and I'm very gentle with myself when I know it needs to be felt.

> **Journal Prompt: What do I think about how my body is responding to exercise during menopause?**

I'm not a fan. [Bad/Snarky]

I don't like that it's changing. [Bad/Petulant]

I want to go back to the way it used to be. [Bad/Whiny]

I want my old body back. [Bad/Sad]

I can't do the things I want to do. [Bad/Powerless] *Zing*

My shoulders sag immediately and I'm sliding slowly backward, down a hole, down a well, down through a tunnel, down in a cave. Down. Down in slow motion. My stomach sinks, my jaw slackens, my arms and legs are jelly and numb. I'm tiny, insignificant, packed in luggage and sent away. My head is full of smoke and my eyes burn. Everything is gray and unfocused. I'm gray. I'm gone. My fingers and toes are worms, squirmy, they want to hide in the dirt. My body is crumbling slowly. I can hear my heart but it's far away. Everything feels far away and so slow. Noise sounds like I'm inside a tin can.

My brain feels quiet for a long time after coming back up from this one. Not quite calm, but not unpleasant, either. I give myself plenty of time to let the feeling finish processing before looking at my journal again. But when I do, I can see that these are thoughts.

I think I'm not a fan. [Bad/Snarky]

I think I don't like that it's changing. [Bad/Petulant]

I think I want to go back to the way it used to be. [Bad/Whiny]

I think I want my old body back. [Bad/Sad]

I think I can't do the things I want to do. [Bad/Powerless]

And when the understanding dawns that because these are thoughts it means they're all optional, I feel clearer in my head again. These thoughts are unhelpful.

I think I'm not a fan. [Bad/Snarky] UNHELPFUL

I think I don't like that it's changing. [Bad/Petulant] UNHELPFUL

I think I want to go back to the way it used to be. [Bad/Whiny] UNHELPFUL

I think I want my old body back. [Bad/Sad] UNHELPFUL

I think I can't do the things I want to do. [Bad/Powerless] UNHELPFUL

One of my greatest takeaways from doing this work is that I am not powerless at all—because I am capable of *feeling* powerless.

Borrow This (Possibly) Helpful Thought

If this chapter has been particularly difficult for you, in terms of sorting through a lifetime of thoughts about how you shouldn't feel your feelings, be aware that your brain might not be ready for the introduction of a helpful thought just yet. I offer these (possibly) helpful gems not only for immediate use, but as little treasures you can tuck in your mental pocket and pull out when it suits you to examine them. And this thought definitely feels like a treasure to me: **I can feel anything.**

For me, this (possibly) helpful thought creates a feeling of deep self-trust, mingled with the power of being capable. I have years of evidence to support the "truthiness" of this statement, and I love to call it up when I notice myself starting to resist a feeling. Of course I can feel anything—*I already have.*

But how does this thought feel for you? Remember, just because it sounds nice doesn't mean it's helpful for you. It has to feel good! So, if this one brings you confidence, power, groundedness, excitement, or hopefulness, then it's a helpful thought. And if it doesn't feel good, it's unhelpful.

Everything We Learned in This Chapter

- Wanting to be happy all the time is part of the reason you feel bad.

- Arguing with reality creates cognitive dissonance, which takes bad feelings and makes them worse.

- Rather than trying to feel good all the time, allow yourself to feel whatever feelings you have—even the bad ones.

- Feeling (temporarily) worse leads to feeling better overall.

- Feelings are uncomfortable but not actually painful. They are also designed to come and go quickly.

- When you allow your feelings to exist in your body without resistance, you will save yourself time, increase your confidence and self-trust, reduce the difficulty of feeling your feelings in the future, and gain agency over your thoughts.

- Difficult feelings come from unhelpful thoughts.

CHAPTER 8

Your Success Story Is Better Than a Fairy Tale

The Honest Story of How to Get Your Goal

A lot of us come to weight loss expecting to achieve it the same way as other goals. You may have followed a simple method, such as the SMART technique of picking something specific, measurable, actionable, reasonable and timebound, and then—*boom!*—goal achieved. Some goals really are that easy! Sure, there may be the occasional setback or point of frustration, but it's not that tough to get what you want. It feels really good to set and smash achievable goals. And I highly recommend that you—at least occasionally—set yourself a goal that requires more from you, in the form of mindset work. Because it feels even better.

Many years ago, when I was still in my thirties, I lost thirty-five pounds with very little trouble. It took me "a long time" (yes, I know that's a thought, and if I'd had it repeatedly while I was losing weight, it certainly would have been unhelpful), but I had almost no mental drama while getting to my goal weight because I'd done it several times before. Truth be told, I white-knuckled my way through the whole nine months and didn't learn a single thing about myself, other than that I apparently had enough willpower to push through hunger, deprivation, and not loving myself very much.

Oh my, did I have a self-awareness bomb waiting for me. As I was nearing my weight-loss goal, I decided to take up running. Suddenly, I was in the thick of nonstop, all day every day, coming at me from all sides, *Drama*.

Every terrible thing I'd ever thought about myself, my ability to follow through, my athletic capabilities, and who I was as a human being (unworthy, unlikable, weird, and stupid) came bubbling to the surface and demanded to be acknowledged. I fumbled my way around with these thoughts for years without getting much agency over them. I set running goals for myself and either missed them by a long shot or—on one heartbreaking occasion—by hundredths of a second. It was ugly, it was painful, and there were a lot of tears. I tried and failed significantly more times than I succeeded.

And yet, I kept coming back for more. Every time I set a new goal for myself to reach a new distance or run faster, I gained the tiniest bit more self-awareness. The process was agonizingly slow—because this was before I started doing intentional mindset work—but undoubtedly worth it. Over the course of nearly two decades of setting my own running, business, and lifestyle goals, I've been through all of the mental drama and made it to the other side.

The great news is that getting one goal is like getting any goal—the same roadblocks, pitfalls, and minefields exist for all of them, and the same success awaits you. **If you have ever achieved any goal in your lifetime, you can achieve every goal you could possibly want.** Your automatic, unmanaged thoughts are the only thing standing in your way, and now you have the Two-Step Tool to get you where you want to go.

There are five inevitable milestones that you'll hit on your way to success. Notably, these unavoidable milestones are applicable to your journey whether you are managing your mind or not. There's no escaping the mental drama just because you know how to journal, and you're not doomed to failure if you're not already finding your thoughts and deciding if they're helpful. But using the Two-Step Tool can help you see your way through the roadblocks faster and more clearly.

I call this process the Get Your Goal Formula, and I like to picture the steps as though they form a check-mark rather than the traditional straight arrow up to your goal. Your first steps into goal-getting work are almost definitely going to feel like you're descending into a deep, dark pit! Then, when you're in the pit you'll hit rock bottom. I know I'm not really selling you here, but it's true, it's unavoidable, and having this information beforehand will help! Finally, beyond rock bottom is where you'll start to climb up, not just to the success you thought you'd have, but well beyond. Truly, the self-awareness you'll gain from your trip into the depths will bounce you up higher than you can imagine right now.

In this chapter, you don't have to just take my word for it. I'll share inspiring real-life stories from some of the clients I've worked with over the years in my group coaching program. These amazing women have walked the check-mark path of the Get Your Goal Formula (some of them long before I gave it that name) and not only lived to tell the tale but are on their way to fulfilling other exciting goals after getting to their desired weight.

The Get Your Goal Formula: Inevitable Success for Every Goal

These are the five milestones you'll reach on your way to achieving your goals.

1. Starting where you are right now and knowing what you want to get

2. Understanding how to get started and choosing a plan

3. Finding more unhelpful thoughts and feelings than you wanted

4. Resisting your goal, even as you're achieving it

5. Knowing who you really are and getting what you want

Milestone 1: Starting where you are right now and knowing what you want to get

This first milestone starts with a wave of excitement and motivation— "I'm going to lose weight once and for all. This is happening!"—that is the brilliant catalyst for change. Even though the phrasing of this milestone makes it sound like you're going to feel clear and precise— almost like putting coordinates into your GPS—for so many women it is marked with confusion, frustration, procrastination, self-doubt, and self-pity.

On the one hand, you know you have weight to lose, you feel like you're ready to do something about it, and you definitely want to lose it. But on the other hand, there's so much information out there about the "best way" to lose weight, and so many people who make it look easy when that's not been your experience, and you're not sure if you can do this at all. There's a good chance you're spending your time researching diets, recipes, exercise routines, or weight-loss programs—gathering information rather than putting it to use.

I rarely work with women who are still at this milestone, because one of the hallmarks of being here is that you don't yet realize that you need help. Or you kind of do, but you're so used to muscling your way through—or you assume you're destined to fail—that you're resistant to asking for help. Here's what the frustration, confusion, and "compare and despair" thoughts from Milestone 1 might sound like in your head (from women I've worked with).

I'm trying to turn my negative into a positive outlook on life. Any suggestions on where I should start my new journey? I've spent more money on fad diets than I can count. I just don't know what is the best way to start.

I am trying to understand. I don't get to eat a lot of calories, but it is what I have to eat to lose weight. I struggle with weekends. What if I want a couple glasses of wine or a dessert? It seems there is no room. Basically you have to give up breakfast, but I am having a real challenge doing that and so I am always overeating my calories. What can I do?

I haven't figured out my food plan as of yet, but I need to get moving, this weight has hit me like a ton of bricks! It's frustrating that what I used to do to lose weight no longer works!

I'm super confused. I used to eat very little and, of course, didn't lose weight. Actually gained! Then went on keto, intermittent fasting, portion control. Arrrgh, now you're saying it's easy. You certainly make it look easy, but it's not.

Pahla, let's talk when you're my age (sixty-three) and see if you look the same, as in as lean as you are now. Just sayin'.

Throughout this milestone you'll feel a dizzying mix of hope, determination, confusion, self-pity, and short-term motivation (meaning, the willingness to make lots of changes all at once, but then struggling to stick with any of them). It's a roller-coaster ride that some women hop off right away, but this step is crucial on your journey because there's no complacency. If you felt fine, you wouldn't be compelled to take action.

Yes, it's true that these negative thoughts and feelings are producing actions that are getting you unwanted results, but that doesn't mean you're stuck. Even women who spend years at Milestone 1—studying different eating plans, investing in trainers or nutritionists, losing some weight, but then quitting and starting over from scratch—can make their way to the next stop. There's no such thing as a standard timeline and getting through this part of the process fast doesn't make the rest of it any easier.

If you are here at Milestone 1, you are already on the path to success, and here's what to do today to move forward: Find one thought. Just one. And really, truly recognize it as a thought. Not just in the "yeah, yeah, yeah, but when am I going to feel better, Pahla?" way, but actually let it sink in. You have the power of thought, and you have the superpower of thinking about your thoughts. When you use your superpower on just one thought, you will be taking the first real step toward your goal.

Milestone 2: Understanding how to get started and choosing a plan

Okay, now you're making progress! You've made the decision that you're not just going to keep complaining about your weight (because those are *thoughts*), and you're committing to a plan and seeing it through. This is the milestone that you thought was going to be the toughest back when you were still at Milestone 1 and spinning in confusion, but moving forward with a tried-and-true weight-loss plan like the 5-0 Method means that you know exactly what to do next. (In fact, there are five things to do next—eat the right number of calories, drink the right amount of water, get the right amount of sleep, exercise moderately, and manage your mind with the Two-Step Tool.) The tricky business is that you might find a real disconnect between knowing what to do and actually doing it.

My client Helen came to me with several of the pieces of her weight-loss puzzle already in place. She was great at drinking water and had a nice, moderate exercise habit that she loved. She was pretty good about sleep and had enough familiarity with journaling that it didn't seem like too much trouble. Counting her calories, though, was the sticking point, and the reason she joined my coaching group.

On our first call, she'd already started using an app to track her calories and was averaging close to her target, so we chatted about how to work journaling with the Two-Step Tool into her daily routine. She was optimistic about being able to move forward with it—especially when I suggested starting with just five minutes a day to find her thoughts—and the next time we met she told me how she'd had several great journaling sessions.

A few weeks later, not only was the calorie tracking starting to slide off her radar, but she hadn't journaled since that first week. "This is what always happens," she announced to me, "I start off great, but then I self-sabotage, get discouraged, and quit."

"Do you know that's a *thought*?" I asked. This is my favorite question to ask my clients, especially near the start of working together, when they really don't know that their thoughts are thoughts. It's so gratifying to watch somebody's mind suddenly open up to a whole new world of possibility.

She was quiet for a moment, and then finally asked, "It's a *thought* that I self-sabotage?"

"Yep," I replied. "Your brain is taking in factual information—you tracked your calories five of the last twelve days and journaled three times in that same period—and then it's telling you a story. You could choose to see those facts as evidence that you're on your way to success, too. 'Self-sabotage' is just a thought, and it's not the only one available to you."

Then we worked through the Two-Step Tool together and she discovered that "I self-sabotage" is an unhelpful thought. And—even more mind-blowing than that—she started to recognize that the feeling of discouragement didn't come from her actions but were created from that thought.

Sometimes the idea that your brain is telling you stories is a lot to take in, particularly if you're new to mindset work. For most of the women I work with, it takes weeks or months of repetition to understand the concept that thoughts and feelings are created in your brain. And beyond that, it can still take months or even years to fully put it into practice in meaningful ways. I don't say this to discourage you! Rather, I hope you take it as reassurance that nothing's wrong with you if you don't "get it" right away. (And, let me be clear: None of this means that you can't lose weight while you're figuring it out.)

Lolly is one of the smartest women I've worked with, and even she struggled to wrestle this idea into her worldview when it came time to decide on a plan for reaching her goal. She had been a member of my group coaching program for months—in fact, she was long past her first goal of weight loss, had already accomplished her second goal of running a half marathon, and was on to her third goal of completing a novel for publication—when she ran into a thought masquerading as a truth: "I don't know what to write."

That thought created such an instantaneous flood of anxiety that of course she wasn't making the kind of progress she wanted to on her novel. The moment she realized that her thought was a thought—and that the anxious feeling was created from her *thought* rather than the act of sitting down in front of her computer to write—was the moment she took a huge leap forward toward her goal. Lolly had understood the concept and put the Two-Step Tool to excellent use many times over. But that day, for that situation, and that thought, and that feeling—it was as if the concept was brand new.

If you are here at Milestone 2 and struggling to put your plan into action, here's how to take the next step forward: Make the connection between your thought and your feeling. Really take the time to detach your feelings from the situations that you once believed was causing them, and recognize them as your own. And once this starts to click—when you're using the Two-Step Tool regularly and have internalized the whole "thoughts create your feelings" thing—you're ready for the next milestone.

Milestone 3: Finding more unhelpful thoughts and feelings than you wanted

Buckle up, friend, because this is where the ride starts to get bumpy! Remember in chapter 2, when you thought, "Oh my goodness, I have a lot of unhelpful thoughts" and I was like, "Yeah," and you wondered, "So, what do I do now?" *This* is what you do now. You keep sorting through them, one by one. And they'll keep coming at you, and you'll keep journaling, and then eventually the tide will turn and you'll be at Milestone 3, where it becomes almost a game to see how many you can find on purpose.

I like to think of this milestone as being where the work goes from the thoughts finding you to you finding the thoughts. When you first got started, it felt like a barrage—thoughts everywhere, just flying at you! But now that you're starting to see them coming from a little farther away, you can put your hand up and catch them with ease. This milestone is where you start to become intentional, which is awesome, and can sometimes be completely overwhelming. Because this is where you start to really take responsibility for your thoughts, learn how to stop beating yourself up for having them, and find out that some of them were hiding even more painful-feeling thoughts underneath them.

Tracey joined my group program because she wanted to lose weight. She'd started and stopped before and was ready to end the struggle once and for all. No sooner did she join the group than it felt like all of our conversations were about her work rather than her weight loss. This is never a problem for me as a coach—all thoughts are thoughts, and they can be recategorized with the Two-Step Tool—and I was curious to see where this exploration would take her.

As it turned out, a lot of the thoughts she was having about work and time management ("There's too much to do" and "I can't get it all done in time") were showing up in her journaling about weight loss, too. Having found and worked through these initial unhelpful thoughts, she had a long stretch of success. For several months, she was on a roll with increased productivity, less stress, and lower numbers on the scale. Then she hit a snag. She knew there were more thoughts to find, and even had some ideas about what they might be, but they eluded her. So, she started looking for them on purpose, in a brilliantly creative way.

Tracey is an incredibly talented artist, and she had noticed that sometimes her brain didn't offer her thoughts directly in words, but they would reveal themselves in her drawings. So, when she arrived here at Milestone 3 and was ready to go searching for those slippery thoughts, she started drawing every day in conjunction with journaling with the Two-Step Tool.

Spending time with her sketchbook and pens before picking up her notebook revealed thoughts she hadn't been able to access through writing alone. And no wonder they had tried to stay under the surface. Tracey's artistic journaling sessions revealed thoughts and feelings that needed to come up and be felt all the way through, no matter the discomfort.

Now, I don't offer you this story to suggest that you have to go and learn how to draw but rather to illustrate that no matter how you come at this work, you can make it your own and be successful with it. There are more thoughts to find than the first dozen or so that present themselves to you, and frankly—they're not going to feel good. That's why they didn't come bubbling up easily.

Annie took a really smart path through this milestone that I love to recommend for anybody who feels overwhelmed by the sheer volume of thoughts that you have in a day that you want to sift through: She decided early on in her weight-loss journey that she would find just three thoughts a day. Her rule is that she never has to do more—unless she wants to in the moment or if the thoughts come to her effortlessly—but she'll also never do less. As it happens, Annie is a fellow endurance runner and also a middle-school math teacher, so she has more experience than most people with breaking unpleasant tasks down into manageable chunks, and a great deal of stick-to-itiveness when the going gets tough.

Within her strict framework of finding three thoughts a day, she allows herself complete freedom—some days she finds thoughts about her husband, or her job, or something she saw on the news, or the number on the scale—and doesn't judge herself for what comes up, even when it's painful or doesn't seem to have an immediate resolution. Annie is internalizing the Two-Step Tool process by practicing it on a wide variety of topics, and as a result, is reaping the benefits in many areas of her life. She knows that it's the practice of finding thoughts and feeling the feelings, rather than the specific thoughts or feelings themselves, that will create amazing changes in her life.

If you are here at Milestone 3 and finding it overwhelming to deal with the number of thoughts, or the intensity of the feelings, here's what to do to move yourself forward: Feel one feeling all the way through. I encourage you to pick the toughest one you can find—the one you've been putting off, the one you think will be the end of you, the one you'd much, much, much rather squirm away from. Once you've tackled it, you'll know the truth: Feelings can't kill you, and—sorry for the cliché, but this one's true—they will make you stronger. And you're going to need access to that strength! This milestone is where the cave starts to look mighty dark, and you'd rather not keep traveling down the steps, but just wait—something even darker is coming next.

Milestone 4: Resisting your goal, even as you're achieving it

Milestone 4 is where you start to access lots of helpful thoughts, and that's *why* it's the hardest and most uncomfortable step of the goal-getting process. I call this milestone "the hard bounce at the bottom" because—particularly while you're down at rock bottom—it's nice to remind yourself that you're going to bounce back out of there. But don't be in a hurry—the bounce is available to you only *after* you've hit the bottom. And sometimes not until you've been flailing around down there for a while.

The hallmark of this milestone is cognitive dissonance—the discomfort you feel when your brain is trying to hold two opposing thoughts at the same time. As you know from chapter 1, your brain does everything in its power to agree with itself, because that's the route of least energy expenditure. But then here you are, starting to recategorize your unhelpful thoughts and think them less often, which leaves room to think your helpful thoughts about your ability to get your goal more often. And those helpful thoughts are in direct opposition to the unhelpful ones, so— yikes! All of a sudden, cognitive dissonance has taken up residence in your brain.

How uncomfortable is cognitive dissonance? Imagine living with a brain that is constantly arguing with itself, because that's *exactly* what's going on. The first time I met Abby she announced to me in no uncertain terms that she was "just always really hard on herself." And she said it as though she was reporting that the sky was blue—as though, *obviously* this was a fact, provable in a court of law, completely unimpeachable, and absolutely unchangeable. "I'm hard on myself" wasn't just a thought in her mind, it was practically a personal mantra.

Then, after she'd been a member of my group for a few months and had met her first goal of losing a hundred pounds, she started realizing that maybe she didn't *have to be* hard on herself. That, in fact, it felt pretty good to be kind to herself, and not only that—but now that she'd been practicing it somewhat regularly, she was getting really good at it.

Well, Abby's brain did not like that one bit, so it doubled down on its efforts to stay efficient. She endured what felt like nonstop self-flagellation and second-guessing for days at a time, and we coached through self-doubt after self-doubt. For months, her brain seemed dead set on blaming her for gaining the weight in the first place and determined to convince her that she didn't know how to lose weight at all. Externally, her weight loss stalled, and internally, she was grappling with hearing thoughts for what they were—*thoughts.*

The tricky thing about this milestone is that both sets of thoughts sound so true! Thankfully, Abby didn't quit on her goal—lots of women do at this stage, because the cognitive dissonance is so uncomfortable, and the unhelpful thoughts trying to keep you from using more energy are *so* painful—and she was able to see what was going on in her brain by using the Two-Step Tool.

Toni came to the group perfectly happy with her weight but frustrated by her eating habits. She had struggled with digestive issues nearly her whole life but couldn't seem to stop, but until she joined the group, she hadn't been able to see the connection with her feelings and thoughts.

During one of our coaching sessions, I guided Toni to think back to the last time she'd eaten something she didn't intend to eat, so we could take a peek at what she'd been thinking, and therefore feeling. She could describe to me what she'd eaten very clearly and had plenty of access to the judgmental thoughts she'd heaped on herself afterward, but she couldn't quite get hold of the thoughts or feelings in the moment of reaching into the cupboard for the food. Thinking that it might help set the scene better, I questioned her about some other details of the day, and finally asked, "When was this?" Her reply: "Oh, this was well over two months ago."

Wait, what?

She'd been living in the reality of her goal—not eating foods that disagreed with her system—for over two months, but she still thought of herself as somebody who struggled to make "good" choices. And when I pointed this out to her, she visibly recoiled. "No, no, no. It's not real yet. This is definitely still a problem" was the response from her efficient, automatic brain. As we talked further and I set her to the task of practicing thinking of herself as successful, I knew I was leading her directly into the hard bounce at the bottom. But—as I've mentioned—it's an *unavoidable* milestone.

Interesting that you can already be at your goal before hitting this milestone, though, right? Your beautiful, efficient brain won't accept new thoughts—even with two months or more of ample evidence—until it has worked through this cognitive dissonance.

Amelia came to group coaching right as she was finishing up her weight-loss journey. She'd had a few bumps along the way, but nothing major, and she felt ready to take on the challenge of maintenance. We spent one or two coaching sessions chatting about her thoughts about the daily tasks she'd continue to do—maintenance comes down to the same five tasks as weight loss: fueling, hydrating, sleeping, exercising, and finding your thoughts to decide if they're helpful—and she took to it in no time at all.

Then she decided she'd like to focus on a work goal. As a salesperson, she has monthly numbers to meet, and she was ready to see if she could stretch a little higher but worried that it would take a lot more work. During our coaching sessions, we talked about how she could work smarter and more efficiently instead of taking more time away from her family. Within a few months, it was obvious that she wasn't just going to meet her goal but that she was going to smash it.

Next, she felt like it was time to tackle something personal that had been bothering her—she wanted to cut down on her drinking habit. She came to this goal full of doubt and worry, but wouldn't you know it, no sooner had she decided exactly what success would look like and created a plan to accomplish it than it was done. She's maintained her moderate drinking protocol for well over a year, at the time of writing of this book.

Watching Amelia sail to goal after goal might seem as though she's not hitting all five of the milestones or, at the very least, that they're not taking her very long. But Amelia's goal-getting streak isn't about achieving any one specific goal—though of course they've all been fantastic—so much as it's about testing how many goals she's "allowed" to have.

After she'd been maintaining her weight for nearly two years, had hit her first big sales goal without working more hours, and cut back on her drinking, Amelia decided she wanted to throw her hat in the ring for a local elected office. Meeting strangers, speaking in public, filling out paperwork, and gathering signatures to get her name on the ballot all seemed to come naturally and easily to her. This looked as though it could be another sure-thing goal to notch in her belt, but I could see that she was finally hitting the hard bounce at the bottom and squirming through cognitive dissonance. She already knew that she could have any goal she wanted. But could she actually have *every* goal she wanted? All of them? Wasn't that greedy?

Of course not, because greedy is a *thought*.

Cognitive dissonance doesn't sound outlandish when it's in your head. It sounds reasonable, and logical, and as if it's the obvious choice for you to make safe decisions and stay in your comfort zone. Cognitive dissonance wants you to keep proving your old thoughts true so you don't use up precious resources on new thoughts. If you feel stranded in the darkness here at Milestone 4, here's how to get through it: Compassionately observe the opposing thoughts of your cognitive dissonance. It is imperative to allow your brain to think what it thinks without believing it, judging yourself for it, arguing back against the thoughts, or trying to force yourself to think positively. When you truly accept that *every* thought you have is just a thought, and you allow the feelings of discomfort to exist without doing something to get rid of them, you're ready to bounce out of here and up to the final stage of success.

Milestone 5: Knowing who you really are and getting what you want

Bouncing out of the bottom doesn't mean that it's *easy* from here on out, but it does get significantly easier at this milestone. Milestone 5 is about waiting out the clock until your goal comes to you (if it hasn't already). Imagine for a moment what it would be like to have absolute certainty that your goal is on its way, and to be living in the reality of having it right now. Your shoulders would relax, your stomach would unclench, and you'd go about your day—because your feelings drive your actions, remember?—like a person who already weighs their goal weight. And you know what a person who weighs their goal weight does? She eats the right amount of food, she drinks the right amount of water, she goes to bed at the same time every night and gets up at the same time every morning, she exercises moderately, and she manages her mind. Just like you, but without the drama.

Jenny was already nearly done losing weight when she joined my coaching group, but like Toni, it took a while for her brain to catch up with her body's changes. When she reached her first weight-loss goal, she immediately set another one of five more pounds, because she felt so sure that it was within reach. And, technically speaking, she could have gotten there if she'd wanted to, but as it turned out, she didn't care that much. Then she worked toward a different fitness goal for a few months, but she didn't quite settle into that one, either.

It wasn't that she wasn't making progress during these "interim" months, though—she was finding thought after thought and feeling *all* of her feelings for the first time in her life. She healed relationships within her family, recognized unhelpful patterns of thinking that had ruled her life, opened herself up to new experiences, and gently dismantled emotional walls that no longer served her.

After a bit of soul-searching—the hard bounce at the bottom—she realized that her body wasn't a goal anymore, but her mind was. So she set out to discover and create her best life, which included the relentless pursuit of fearlessly feeling her feelings. She'd been stuffing them down and trying to ignore them her whole life, and it was time to let them all out and set herself free.

Can you imagine setting yourself a goal to feel all your feelings? Where the daily task is to find your most uncomfortable thoughts and then feel *whatever* comes up? That's what Jenny did, and it's been a wonder to behold.

When you're not afraid of your feelings, you're not afraid of anything.

After a year of living her best life and exploring her thoughts and feelings, Jenny realized that there was another tangible goal to set for herself in business: being seen and creating a new type of success for herself by helping others work through their mindset journey. Because she realized that anybody—*everybody!*—can feel as good about themselves as she does. She is now a certified goal coach, helping women achieve their fitness dreams.

Sharon took nearly five years to lose 115 pounds. She started by eating less, exercising more, and holding herself to the highest standard of perfection for these tasks, as so many of us do. But after she gave herself stress fractures in both ankles at the same time, she knew it was time to try something different, and that's when we started working together.

Even though she understood intellectually that she need to make changes, she resisted them at every turn. Counting calories? No, thank you. Exercising moderately? Ummm, that can't possibly work. And mindset work with a journal? Definitely a hard pass. I believe her exact words were, "No effing way, Pahla!"

I'll confess that I love the "resisters" a little more than my clients who come to me ready to believe everything I say (though of course I love them, too). Part of it is that I'm also a contrarian by nature, and the skeptic in me sees and honors the skeptic in you. Additionally, it's just so dang rewarding for me to watch self-awareness dawn little by little, until one day it's just bright full sunshine, and you *get it*. "Resister" clients like Sharon have to wrestle with the ideas and concepts I teach until they've truly made their own way through. And when that happens, look out, world!

Sharon's weight loss was reasonably steady and marked by weeks and even months of plateaus, but there was never a point where she wasn't making dramatic progress *somewhere* in her life. Even though weight loss was her main focus, she found herself journaling—and finding plenty of unhelpful thoughts—about her relationships with her mother and her son. She found the courage to quit a job that wasn't serving her, grieved the loss of her sister, and confronted decades of old beliefs about what it means to be strong. After a lifetime of not wanting to be weak—which included thoughts like, "I have to be big," "I can't get under two hundred pounds" and "I can't weigh less than a man"—she discovered that it takes more strength to feel through your uncomfortable feelings than to deny them. And when she did, she opened herself up to the exciting possibilities that were waiting behind worry, sadness, anger, and embarrassment.

On the day she reached her weight goal, she shared her joy in the group—allowing herself to be the center of attention, which was another uncomfortable feeling she was willing to feel—and announced her next goal: Easily maintaining her weight for the rest of her life. Because she had learned through her journey that she can do anything she sets her mind to.

> **Journal Prompt: What do I think about success stories?**

Oh, did you think we weren't going to use the Two-Step Tool in this chapter? Well, we are, and I suspect that you're going to find some easily accessible helpful thoughts—that's why we love reading success stories, after all. So here we go. My stated goal, the thing I came to my journal for self-awareness about is "I help women see what's possible for them." These are thoughts that I found.

If they can do it, anybody can.

I love it when people get what they want.

It's possible.

Everybody can do this.

Yes, these are thoughts and I can choose them any time I want to!

I think if they can do it, anybody can.

I think I love it when people get what they want.

I think it's possible.

I think everybody can do this.

And these thoughts create really lovely feelings for me, which means they are definitely HELPFUL.

I think if they can do it, anybody can. [Good/Inspired] HELPFUL

I think I love it when people get what they want. [Good/Generous] HELPFUL

I think it's possible. [Good/Excited] HELPFUL

I think everybody can do this. [Good/Generous] HELPFUL

Even Better Than Happily Ever After

Your story doesn't end the day you get your goal weight, and—as I've made abundantly clear throughout this book—your goal weight won't make you happy. So why do any of this work? Why lose weight, or learn to love yourself, or set new goals for your future?

Because you can.

You are an incredible human being who is worthy and deserving of the things you desire. You are a lovable person who belongs here and is capable of doing anything. You are simultaneously a miracle and a *mess* (sorry, but it's true) because you're supposed to be both. That's just the nature of being human. You have all the power you need because you have the power of your thoughts. And because your thoughts create feelings, you have that power at your fingertips, too.

YOU have the power, the ability, the permission, and the responsibility to live your best life. Your weight? I know it seems important right now, but truly, the significance is in the journey to get your goal—because it will show you everything amazing and brilliant and capable that you have inside of you.

Go get your goal.

ACKNOWLEDGMENTS

This book would still be a "maybe someday" dream in my brain if it weren't for Laurie Y., who wanted to write it for me, and Lori O., who insisted—quite bossily, I might add—that I write it myself. (You were right, of course.)

But even then I didn't go it alone, and thank goodness. Camille Noe Pagan, book and life coach extraordinaire, helped me wrestle with my brain and responded with ALL CAPS ENTHUSIASM when I needed it most.

Michele Martin, you are a terrific, tenacious agent, and it's been so reassuring to have your guidance on this publishing adventure— thanks for being by my side.

Many, many thanks to the entire team at The Experiment for welcoming me so warmly and helping me create a book even better than I thought I could. In particular, thank you to Batya Rosenblum for your gentle, insightful editing. You took this manuscript from pretty darn good to literally amazing (this sentence is killing you, isn't it?), and I'm so grateful for every red line. Besse Lynch, thank you for coordinating publicity and being as excited to promote the book as I am. And, oh my goodness, thank you to Beth Bugler for knocking my socks off with such a bold, powerful cover design.

To all of my beautiful Bs on YouTube, thank you! Who knew that an awkward 15-minute balance ball video could turn into *all this*?

My GYG friends, who are each a circumstance about whom I have many thoughts that create feelings of delight—your support, your questions (because that's how we show love), your curiosity, and your willingness to persevere through vulnerability are nothing short of awe-inspiring. You make me a better coach and a better human being, and I'm so grateful for every one of you.

They probably thought I was weird kid for loving to play with the typewriter as much as any toy, but my parents encouraged me to find my own way in the world. Thank you, Mom and Dad, for knowing I was going to be a writer one day.

Thank you always to Mike, who takes the role of big brother very seriously and does it so well. I'm lucky to have you, as was Vicki.

To my wonderful boys, Andy and Jake—thanks for listening to your mom talk about menopause so much.

All my love to my Davey B, who put up with long stretches between haircuts and quiet evenings alone while I was writing. Thank you for listening while I verbally reorganized entire chapters, even when you had no idea what I was talking about, for finishing the laundry I always forgot (even when I'm not writing a book), and for being the best adventure buddy a girl could ask for. P heart D forever.

ABOUT THE AUTHOR

PAHLA BOWERS is a certified weight-loss life coach for women over 50, with over a decade of experience helping women make peace with their menopausal bodies. She is the host of the *Get Your GOAL* podcast and a prolific online content creator with expertise in women's health, personal development, and menopause fitness. *Mind Over Menopause* is her first book. She lives in California.

You can find her at getyourgoal.com.

 PahlaB

pahlab_weightlosscoach

pahla_b

PahlaB

The B Hive